*MAKING A DIFFEREN*

*HUMAN HORIZONS SERIES*

# MAKING A DIFFERENCE IN CANCER CARE

*Practical Techniques in
Palliative and Curative Treatment*

## CLARE RUSHWORTH

*A Condor Book
Souvenir Press (E&A) Ltd*

First published 1994 by Souvenir Press
(Educational & Academic) Ltd,
43 Great Russell Street, London WC1B 3PA
and simultaneously in Canada

ISBN 0 285 63215 9

Printed in Great Britain by
The Guernsey Press Co. Ltd, Guernsey, Channel Islands

*This book is dedicated to my son, Simon,*
*who is always ready to help; and to my*
*husband, Darrell, who is without doubt*
*'the wind beneath my wings'*
*(which is no mean feat!)*

# Foreword

Cancer medicine is undergoing a quiet revolution. In part this is due to the development of multidisciplinary patterns of care and a recognition that the best standards draw on the expertise of all types of carer. It is our duty to learn new skills where necessary and to improve those we already have. I must admit to having been rather sceptical of these techniques before meeting Clare. My experience has now shown that they work. This book shows recognisable aspects of our own and our patients' behaviour. You may be surprised to discover that you are already practising some of the psychological techniques discussed in this book. To look at these methods through Clare's eyes is to allow yourself to harness them in a new way; an expert guide transforms a pleasant country walk into a rich experience by pointing out details and delights that would otherwise have remained unnoticed.

An important feature of *Making a Difference in Cancer Care* is that it allows patients to regain an element of control over the situation in which they find themselves. The best test of any professional is to ask to whom the other staff go for help. I don't like heights!! I still don't like heights. The difference is that after talking to Clare I can get nearer the edge of a cliff!

In *Alice in Wonderland*, Alice asked the Cheshire Cat, 'Would you tell me, please, which way I ought to go from here?' 'That depends a good deal on where you want to get to,' said the Cat. 'I don't much care where—' said Alice. 'Then it doesn't matter which way you go,' said the Cat. For all of us involved in looking after patients with cancer, be it with curative or palliative intent, it does matter which 'way' we go. This book will lead you in the right direction.

Adrian Crellin

# Contents

# Acknowledgements

When I am asked how long it took me to learn the skills I teach in this book, my apparently flippant answer is 'Forty-five years.' As long as I can remember I have had an insatiable curiosity about what makes people tick, and about the power of the human mind. During the last fifteen years or so, however, I have been able to focus my efforts and have had the opportunity to learn things that I found amazing, from some wonderful people who, like me, are blessed (or cursed?) with curiosity.

Dr Lawrence Le Shan taught me to meditate; Wilf Proudfoot was responsible not only for teaching me to be a hypnotherapist, but for providing me with my first 'jaw-dropping' experiences of neuro-linguistic programming. From Robert Dilts, one of the pioneers and developers of NLP, I learned about 'belief systems and health'. While having a whale of a time doing my NLP master practitioner course with Ian McDermott of International Teaching Seminars, I encountered John Hicks, brilliant teacher and human being. Also during this period I became proficient in time line therapy, a branch of NLP, with Tad James.

Then there are those who believe in me: Dr Sheila Cartwright, consultant in radiotherapy and oncology, who 'discovered' me several years ago and gave me the chance to show what I could do and the leeway to do it; Mavis Robinson, Macmillan nurse, who seems to be the only person who realises when I am overdoing things (she says I get 'cross')—however, because she incessantly sings my praises as a therapist and trainer I keep having to overdo things; the palliative care team at St James's University

Hospital in Leeds, who keep asking me back to teach, as do Frank Couling of the Marie Curie Education Centre in London and the tutors at various hospice study centres—to them my thanks for providing me with opportunities to develop my fairly 'off the wall' style of teaching; and my friends from the ITS class of '93, who encouraged me to write this book—John Lavan, Mariella Cook, Colin Blundell, Dr John Phillips, Allan Unnuck, Dr Brian Gough and Helen Connolly.

Of course, none of it would have been possible without my patients, who constantly amaze me with their courage and their willingness to go along with my, sometimes bizarre, ideas.

In many ways I have kept the best until last. There are three people without whom this book would never have been more than an idea, and much of the credit for it should go to them: my husband (who was my cartoonist) and son, who have given me time, space, encouragement, love and total support, not only throughout the writing of this book but whenever I have needed it; and Penny Parks, amazing human being, author, trainer, also of the class of '93, who has supported this project right from its inception with unstinting love, advice and encouragement—thank you for being my friend.

C.R.

# Introduction

This is a practical book, a book specifically aimed at those working with people with cancer—although the information and techniques can equally well be applied in any area of health care. It has evolved from my work with countless people who have the disease and from my training sessions for health care professionals, and it sets out my approach to helping people deal with their diagnosis, prognosis and symptoms, and the side-effects of any treatment. Above all, this book derives from my belief that it is always possible, in some way or other, to make a difference in the life of a person dealing with what is probably his or her worst nightmare—cancer.

People with no experience of working in the field of cancer care often give me 'that look' that you have probably seen yourself. They look at me dewy-eyed and say something like, 'I don't know how you can do your job. Don't you get upset [sad/depressed]? I couldn't do it!' If you have ever watched the spoof disaster movie, *Airplane*, you will have seen 'that look' on the faces of the passengers when the nun sings a song to the sick child . . . When I tell them that I would break in at night to do my work if no one would employ me to do it, when I tell them that I have a horror of my employers discovering that what I do is not 'work', when I try to tell them how much I love what I do—they begin to look perplexed, as if I am something from another planet.

Sometimes the look intensifies, as if they have stumbled on Mother Teresa—you have probably had that happen too. Then I attempt to explain that if someone is ill, needs help or is frightened, and you would really like to help but cannot . . . it is *then* that you feel helpless, at a loss, sad . . . or even distraught. But if you *can* in some way make things easier for that person, if you *can* help, if you can *make a difference* in his or her life, then you will feel an incredible 'buzz' and a profound sense of satisfaction. In my own case, it is at times like this that I believe I am justifying my existence.

If you are reading this book, then it is almost inevitable that you know exactly what I am talking about. In my experience, the health care professionals who are looking for new or better ways to help their patients—the ones reading the books and taking the courses—are the ones who are already doing a brilliant job. It is the people who believe that they already know all there is to know about dealing with patients who should be reading this. So, in a sense, I am already preaching to the converted, the ones who are making a difference already. Here I invite you to share some of the things I too have learned (and am still learning) about making a difference in the lives of our patients. Along the way you will also learn techniques that are applicable to the rest of your life, to yourself . . . because I believe that in order to care for others we need to have a caring attitude towards ourselves.

The techniques in this book are drawn from a variety of disciplines and are all aimed at reducing stress, restoring some measure of control in, and improving, the lives of people dealing with cancer. This includes those having curative or palliative treatment (often these fields overlap) and those just living with the disease. Simply reducing stress has beneficial implications both physically and emotionally, in areas such as anxiety, pain control, appetite and digestion, energy and sleeping. These are fully discussed in Chapter 1.

Although I had a grounding in nursing and social work, I have spent much of the latter part of my life in learning how our minds work and about using the mind to our benefit. If you have ever read Terry Pratchett's hilarious Discworld novels you might recall that one of his characters, Granny Weatherwax, practises what she calls 'headology'. I would like to be Granny Weatherwax when I grow up, with her blend of pragmatism, curiosity, common sense and practical experience. I am proud to practise headology! Incidentally, when patients ask me, 'Is there anything I should be reading?' (usually meaning books on cancer), I often reply, 'Yes, Terry Pratchett.' Laughter is extremely beneficial for both mind and body.

Under the banner of 'headology' I include techniques drawn from neuro-linguistic programming, hypnosis, meditation and relaxation. Neuro-linguistic programming (NLP) is 'state of the art' in the fields of therapy and communication. Developed in the 1970s by Richard Bandler and John Grinder, NLP is about how we communicate—consciously and unconsciously—with others; and with ourselves (that is, how we think). It is about how we shape our reality, and consequently how that reality affects us physically and emotionally. Tad James gives the following definition of NLP:

*Neuro*—The nervous system (the mind), through which our experience is processed via five senses: visual, auditory, kinesthetic, olfactory, gustatory.

*Linguistic*—Language and other non-verbal communication systems through which our neural representations are coded, ordered and given meaning. Includes: pictures, sounds, feelings, tastes, smells, words (self-talk).

*Programming*—The ability to discover and utilise the programs that we run (our communication to ourselves and others) in our neurological systems to achieve our specific and desired outcomes.

In other words, NLP is how to use the language of the mind consistently to achieve our specific and desired outcomes.

I could go on endlessly about NLP and its uses in communicating, training, self-development . . . In this book you will find out how to use NLP techniques to gain rapport easily, quickly and consistently with patients (and people in general); how to heighten your sensitivity to patients' non-verbal communication; and how to relax them while getting on with your routine work. You will find out how to deal with phobias and traumas simply, gently, respectfully and painlessly; and discover a little of how we structure our reality and how this knowledge can be used.

You will learn techniques to use with patients for their well-being: simple relaxation methods which take up little time but can have a profound effect on their state, some to talk them through and others to teach them for their own use. I would almost always rather teach than 'therap', as patients often feel that their life went out of their control with the diagnosis. Giving them techniques which they can use to improve their own well-being can immediately reduce stress and helplessness.

Meditation can be a most effective way of reducing stress, with all the subsequent benefits to emotional and physical well-being, as well as a way of learning to live more fully 'in the now'. I offer a variety of methods of meditation which, alongside the techniques derived from self-hypnosis, will not conflict with any religious beliefs a patient may hold. None of these methods are in any way attempts at 'mind-emptying' (for my views on this topic see Chapter 3). Contrary to popular belief, hypnosis does not require a swinging watch. Whenever we imagine or remember anything vividly we are in a light trance similar to that induced by hypnosis—as in that blissful state just before drifting off to sleep, or when we almost miss our exit on the motorway. Hypnosis is about an altered state of awareness focused internally rather than externally.

In my training sessions I include the material presented in this book, but in a deliberately different format. Here there are separate chapters on topics such as meditation and relaxation, and each chapter covers several methods. If I were to follow this pattern while training—if I did all the relaxation techniques one after another—then, whatever topic followed, I would be unlikely to get much sense out of anyone. Similarly, although while training I have to continually change pace and subject, to do this in a book could make for difficult reading (and lots of tiny chapters). Here, then, you will find that each chapter covers a specific area, with one exception: over the years I have collected various techniques, to help patients, which do not fit neatly under a single heading, and these I have bunched together in the final chapter.

I explore here what may well be unfamiliar territory for you, and so I have assumed that you have no prior knowledge in any of the techniques. I have also assumed that you have very little spare time to apply them! There are, however, some simple guidelines to their successful use.

First, allow yourself a little time to master the techniques; read and re-read until you are clear about what to do. Second, it is essential to be congruent—that is, to *act as if* you expect the methods to work. Some of the techniques may seem bizarre, until you have tried them and been successful, so you may feel hesitant when using them. If you appear doubtful to your patients, this will not help you to achieve your aim, which is to do something that benefits them—that makes a difference in their life. So, *act as if* you know exactly what you are doing and why you are doing it; believe in yourself and your good intentions. With a few successes under your belt you will find that you no longer have to act. Remember, though, that nothing terrible will happen if you do not get it right first time!

These are powerful techniques, drawn from the best in their respective fields, so please use them with respect, love and, above all, *a sense of humour*. I hope I will succeed in giving you the flavour of my training courses—in which you will find, of course, all the formal aims and objectives that you would expect, but also my other, poorly hidden, agenda: that everyone shall enjoy him- or herself hugely while learning some amazing stuff! As you will discover when you read on, with this book and your goodwill you can make a difference in all manner of ways. Not only will you be able to help your patients sleep well, be in control, have less pain, regain their appetites, get the best from their treatment, but, most importantly—whatever their diagnosis and prognosis—you will be able to help them to *live*.

# 1 The Stress Spiral

One definition of stress is anything you have to adapt to. A patient has symptoms, then medical staff subject him to X-rays, blood tests, endoscopies, bronchoscopies and so forth. He may have to be admitted to hospital, where he has to adapt to a strange bed, hospital food, changing staff, maybe more tests; possibly surgery, chemotherapy or radiotherapy. There is a diagnosis, a prognosis—possibly poor—forcing changes in future plans, dreams and hopes. Relationships may become a problem, as patient and family have to adapt to changing roles. A husband and breadwinner may become a dependent invalid, at home all the time. A career woman, used to making decisions and being in control of her life, can suddenly find that the most important part of her life, her health, is in someone else's hands (albeit temporarily). Then there may be pain, nausea, anorexia and a multitude of other troubles caused by the illness—as well as other problems in the patient's life. All these things, and more, he or she has to adapt to and deal with.

## THE FIGHT-OR-FLIGHT RESPONSE

As long as we have been on earth we have had the **fight-or-flight response** to help us deal instantly with potential threats. This response was intended to deal with short-term physical threats such as wild animals or a man attacking with a club. After the threat had been dealt with, and assuming our ancestor was still alive, the parasympathetic nervous system moderated the fight-or-flight response until next time. Unfortunately, even now we have not developed

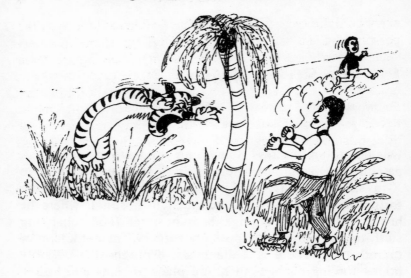

*The fight-or-flight response.*

any other way of dealing with threats, and we still respond to *any* problem by getting ready to fight or run. Difficulties arise when the threat is not one that can be dealt with in this way, such as illness, or financial or relationship problems, where the signal to 'stand down' never comes; or when the threats come one after the other over a long period.

If we look at some of the changes brought about by the fight-or-flight response in both the short and the long term, you will begin to see why I place such great emphasis on reducing patients' stress, and how using and teaching the techniques in this book can make a vital difference to the well-being of your patients. What I am about to describe is a model of what happens in stress—a simplified model, certainly, but if you **act as if** it were a true picture then you will go a long way to understanding what happens to stressed people.

Initially, the fight-or-flight response releases endorphins, the body's own painkillers; this reaction to danger came about so that if our ancestor was bitten or injured he could carry on fighting or running. We have all heard stories of the person who, having his leg ripped off by a combine harvester, crawls on hands and remaining knee across three fields and phones for the ambulance. This is partly thanks to endorphins. However, in long-term stress endorphins are depleted and the patient has a lowered pain threshold and so needs more medication—with the obvious possibility of drug-related problems such as constipation, drowsiness, nausea and confusion.

## Physical problems caused by stress

When the threat is perceived, muscles tense—after all, you cannot fight or run with relaxed muscles. This muscle tension can lead to increased pain, or cause it where there was previously none. It is a fairly common occurrence for people to be admitted to hospital with suspected meningitis or coronary problems, when the real cause is stress-related muscle tension. Most health care professionals will be aware of the **pain cycle** of someone with severe pain (see diagram 1): pain already experienced generates a fear of pain to come, which in turn generates tension, which brings on more pain, and so on.

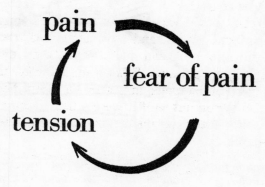

*The pain cycle.*

There are thus three components of pain—remembered pain, actual pain and anticipated pain—so depleted endorphins and muscle tension will, in time, increase the severity of each of these. In preparation for fighting or running, digestion is repressed as the blood supply from stomach and bowels is diverted to brain and limbs. If you have ever suffered from 'butterflies' before an interview, then you have experienced this happening. Long-term, this can lead to indigestion (or even ulcers), diarrhoea, constipation or anorexia. And it can become an emotive issue, as well-meaning carers try to encourage the patient to eat the meals that they have lovingly prepared.

Often carers feel helpless, and feeding the patient is one of the ways in which they *can* feel useful (after all, 'as long as he's eating, there can't be much wrong with him, can

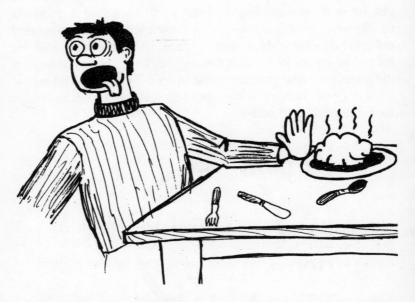

*In preparation for fight or flight, the blood supply from stomach and bowels is diverted to brain and limbs—which can lead, in the long term, to chronic indigestion or anorexia.*

there?'). If the patient does try to force the food into an unwilling digestive system, the result is nausea and indigestion. Add this to the nausea, taste changes and other eating problems that can be caused by some types of chemotherapy and radiotherapy, and there can be severe difficulty in maintaining weight and energy. Salivary glands, being part of the digestive system, also turn off during threat. As a sore, dry mouth can be a result of some cancer treatment, lack of saliva is an added problem in chewing and swallowing.

Just as a car engine has to be cooled to run efficiently, so sweating occurs to cool the muscles as they burn their fuel to produce energy. Unfortunately, this is a little like leaving the engine running while your car is standing in the drive, or leaving your central heating on with the door and windows open. It is a complete waste of energy, and people in long-term stress will often be chronically tired, adding to the lack of energy that may be a result of their disease, treatment, loss of appetite or insomnia. Furthermore, heart rate and respiration increase so as to carry more oxygenated blood to the limbs and brain. Long-term, this can lead to arrhythmia, blackouts and breathing problems. People suffering from stress often yawn or sigh frequently, so the problems for someone with existing respiratory difficulties are obvious. Initially in the fight-or-flight response, cortisone is released as an aid in keeping the airways open—after all, it is not conducive to survival to have an allergy or asthma attack while running away from your attacker; and this *is* what the fight-or-flight response is meant to deal with. Dyspnoea causes stress, and stress increases respiratory problems. Anticipating the need to deal with possible injury, fibrinogen is released and blood vessels constrict so that the blood will clot more easily at the site of any wound that may be inflicted.

Another reaction to threat is the release of sugar into the circulation as fuel for limbs and brain; this has an effect on energy levels and moods—and not only for people with diabetes. Cholesterol is also released to help the muscles use the fuel efficiently; combine this with increased heart rate, thickened blood ready to clot and narrowed blood vessels, and you have raised blood pressure—and a ticking time-bomb!

In the long term, the immune system can become compromised. Have you ever found that when you are 'run down' (another euphemism for 'stressed') you seem to pick up bugs from anyone within a mile of you?

These are just *some* of the potential physical problems.

## Emotional and psychological difficulties caused by stress

It may help to set the scene if you imagine how it would be if you found yourself in a tiger-infested forest. An individual who has had a lot of problems that could not be dealt with by fighting or running, so that they were never really resolved; who has continuing difficulties (as with patients); and who has possible future problems, is in the twentieth-century equivalent of the tiger-infested forest. There are the

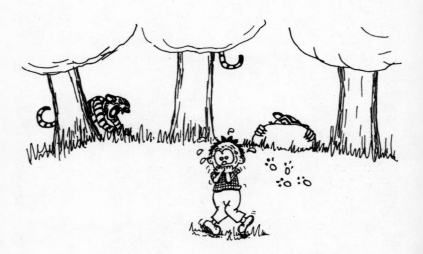

*How would it be in a tiger-infested forest?*

'tigers' that are the memories of past problems, diagnoses, tests; of being given 'the news', of treatment, and of family reactions . . . all the things that have had to be adapted to. There are the current 'tigers' in that individual's life, which could include treatment, emotional problems—a thousand and one things that may be happening to him now. Then there are the future 'tigers': all the worries about what might or might not happen, how the treatment is going, and what might happen to him and his family if it does not go well.

The problem here is that remembered and imagined 'tigers' might as well be current ones: we react to what our minds are focusing on, whether real or imagined. Just for a few moments remember, as vividly as you can, a time when you were scared; or if you have a phobia, focus on the object of that phobia . . . How do you feel? Before going any further, remember a time of joy, laughter or triumph . . . Now you may proceed.

So someone having to deal with cancer is often in the situation of having to function in the equivalent of the tiger-infested forest—registering that his survival is threatened from many directions. And when our survival is threatened, all our resources are directed at dealing with the threats.

Even when a person is diagnosed and given an excellent prognosis, he can hear the word 'cancer', or something with 'oma' at the end of it, and temporarily react as if his future is no longer than the distance to the end of his nose. Imagine that you have had symptoms for which you have had a series of tests: you are already seeing 'tigers' in your mind's eye because you have problems and cannot yet fix them. Then you are told that you have cancer. You now know the size of the tiger because you know of lots of people—acquaintances, film and sports stars—who got cancer and died! At this point people often stop listening. It can be quite some time before they can be emotionally convinced that the tigers can be dealt with. Intellectually they may know that 'if I had to get cancer then this was the best sort to get. I've been one of the lucky ones.' You have probably heard this yourself from patients. But the emotional realisation takes longer; after all, this *is* the survival instinct at work. Our ancestors that yawned and said, 'Sabre-toothed tiger . . . so what?' probably got eaten—so they are probably *not* our ancestors anyway (or anyone else's!).

I recently worked with a young woman who had been told she had lymphoma. Fortunately it had been diagnosed at a very early stage, and her prognosis could not have been much better. Her treatment was not particularly unpleasant and, apart from a little tiredness, she had no physical problems. Her consultant, having given her the diagnosis and prognosis, was completely nonplussed when she became distressed, and kept repeating to her mother and to the nurse, 'But I'm giving her *good* news!' As I said, even those with a good prognosis often take a while to emotionally accept it.

Initially in the fight-or-flight response, the senses and reactions become sharper—you need to be alert if you are in an area where you believe there are tigers! Long-term, these heightened senses scanning for threats can cause problems with intolerance to noise and other stimuli. This state can also lead to a form of free-floating anxiety, as the brain attempts to make sense of the physiological stress signals it is receiving. The patient has been stressed for some time, but probably nothing particular is happening at this moment. However, registering stress and trying to make sense of the signals, the brain concludes that there *must* be a potential threat somewhere around. Have you ever had that feeling of impending doom, that *something* is about to happen? Well, by the law of averages sometimes something *will* go wrong, and that is when you think you have had a premonition. We tend not to remember all the times that we have had this feeling of vague anxiety and nothing has happened.

Patients can become stuck in their anxiety and appear to be looking for problems, or exaggerating minor ones. Remember, we are dealing with the survival instinct here, and no one ever got eaten by *over*estimating the size of the tiger.


## OUR PERCEPTION OF REALITY

Imagine, for a moment, that you have ordered a new car—for example, a red Fiesta—and you are going to collect it tomorrow. It is a fair bet that suddenly every other car on the road appears to be . . . a red Fiesta. This is because our brains **filter** information coming at us; we could not function if we had to pay attention to absolutely everything, so we focus on what is important currently. Having said that, even the things that we do allow through our filters are not necessarily an accurate representation of reality, and this can lead to even more stress. A look at a simplified version of the neuro-linguistic programming communication model might be helpful at this point (see diagram 2), to illustrate what happens to 'reality' before we make sense of it, and how this can affect people's behaviour, and their physical and emotional states. This in turn helps us to understand why patients (and people in general) sometimes appear to be acting irrationally. If we can gain a measure of insight into the internal process that is going on, then we are in a much better position to help them reach a more resourceful state.

*We do not have direct contact with 'reality'*. By the time we have registered that something has happened, and made sense of it, we are already remembering it—if only at a split second's remove. We do not have two holes in the front of our heads with a *direct* view of the world, nor do we have two holes at the side of our heads that *directly* receive sound. When an event occurs, the image on the retina is encoded through the optic nerves and decoded in a specific part of the brain. Similarly, when soundwaves hit the eardrum they are encoded, then decoded in the brain. It is the same with sensations carried along other nerves. So, by the time we have gathered and collated information from our senses, and made some sense of it, the moment has already passed. It is a little like a TV outside broadcast transmission where the camera and microphone take in pictures and sounds, encode them and then transmit the signals to your television, which decodes the signals so that you can receive the images and sounds on the screen.

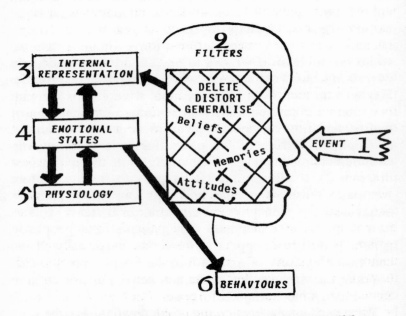

*The neuro-linguistic programming communication model.*

Unlike the outside broadcast, however, humans do not decode directly what was received and transmitted from the outside world. We are meaning-making animals, and our brains process the 'broadcast' before it is played on our internal TV. Our brains do this to help us survive; to prevent us from making the same mistakes over again and from having to keep re-learning things—so that we can actually function in the world. Back to diagram 2: the *event* (1) is seen, heard, felt, smelled and tasted; then it is passed through various *filters* (2) to make meaning from what is being received.

These filters delete, distort and generalise our experiences so that they fit in with what we already 'know' about the world. The filters can be created from our memories, experiences, culture, beliefs and many other things. When we are young we learn how to recognise and operate a door, and this soon generalises to all doors, no matter what size, colour or type of handle. If this were not the case, we would get locked in every time we found ourselves in a strange room with a closed door! We generalise so that we do not have to spend all our lives working out how to do simple things over and over. Imagine how it would be if you recognised a chair only if it were a replica of your first chair; or if you had not generalised that *all* people who rapidly go bluish probably need help immediately! Generalising usually makes life easier. Unfortunately, sometimes it causes problems.

I was asked to see one woman who, every time she was approached by someone in a white coat, panicked and became incontinent. This was obviously distressing for my patient, as well as degrading, and was making it difficult for doctors to help her. They could probably have improved matters by removing their coats, but there was always the chance that someone would forget or that the patient would be transferred elsewhere and the problem would recur.

A little history-taking revealed that this person had never, until the previous two weeks, been in hospital. At that point she had been admitted to a teaching hospital because of breathing difficulties and haemoptysis. It had obviously been a traumatic experience for her, and part of that experience had been that she was surrounded by a group of people (consultant with retinue) in white coats. It was one of these people in a white coat who eventually told her that she had inoperable cancer of the lung. The mind learns very quickly, and much more rapidly during traumatic times. On this occasion her brain learned and generalised that all people in white coats bring terrifying news. Her mind had done a brilliant, instant, but mistaken job of learning that day. From then on she did not have to go to the trouble of consciously remembering what she had learned—it went straight into her unconscious mind, which could reproduce the terror instantly at the sight of a white coat. Participants on my courses often laugh when I remark on what an amazing skill it is to be able to learn something like this so rapidly and completely that you *never* forget to do it. People would pay good money for a skill like that! So you can see how generalising might affect our perception of reality. The good news is that I was able, in this instance, to remedy the problem simply and painlessly with a technique that you will find later in the book (see p. 138).

To return to our 'filters': portions of a communication can get deleted because, for instance, of a belief that 'everyone who gets cancer dies'. As with the young woman with lymphoma, any evidence that conflicts with this 'belief filter' is unlikely to get through. Patients often tell me, 'Every magazine and newspaper I pick up and every television programme I see has something about cancer in it!' Logically, we know this cannot be true. If it *were* true, publishers and television companies would not stay in business for long; but because these patients are currently under threat from the disease, they have set in motion a 'cancer filter' which allows through information on the subject, but not amusing or distracting things.

The meaning of communications from the outside world can become distorted because of these filters. If patients feel that they have been misinformed by other health care professionals in the past, or if they have been given a diagnosis that subsequently turned out to be wrong, then they will have a 'mistrust filter'. This could provoke in them, as a first reaction, the conviction that any future information given will be, at worst, a lie and at best not to be relied on.

There are many filters that change the meaning of an event before we make sense of it, but, whatever the filter, the result is that we play an edited version of reality on our 'inner screen'—our *internal representation* (3, in diagram 2). It is this version of reality that we react to, leading to an *emotional state* (4)—this could be terror, anxiety, pleasure, relief, joy or any one of the whole gamut of feelings which humans are capable of, depending on whatever 'movie' we are currently showing in our heads.

This emotional state in turn affects our *physiology* (5); it could activate the fight-or-flight response, or induce relaxation, or whatever. If you have a patient who is sitting slumped, staring at the floor and sighing, it is a fair assumption that her internal movie—what she is thinking—is not full of fun and joy. If, for instance, it is the fight-or-flight response that has been triggered, then the physiological state (as discussed earlier) will feed back to the emotions, raising the anxiety further. The emotional state will then lead to certain *behaviours* (6), conscious and unconscious: anger or agitation, for example, or the sudden inability to take in information or, sometimes, apparently irrational behaviour.

I believe that an individual's behaviour is always rational, even if the reason is not immediately clear to us. He is simply reacting to *his* inner representation of the world (as we all do), and the only reason that he appears to the rest of us to be acting or thinking irrationally is that we have a different representation of reality. This different representation of reality will coincide in some ways with that of the majority of people (in which case we are considered 'sane'), but in many ways it will not as we have not got their filters. This is why I believe it is crucial, if we wish to help patients, to try to understand as far as possible the meaning they are making of what is happening to them. Then, rather than giving them what we merely *think* they need, we have a better chance of actually communicating and helping effectively. For people in the caring professions it is also a great stress-proofer if, rather than getting frustrated or upset at a patient's behaviour (as we all do at times, because we too are human!), we can remember that patients have a different map of reality from ours. One thing I always try to bear in mind is that people in 'not normal' situations can often be expected to act 'not normally'!

So, back in the tiger-infested forest . . . A person in the grip of the fight-or-flight response will focus on threats, ignoring other things, so that gradually his reality changes. If all you are focusing on is problems, real or imagined, imagine how easy it is to progress from anxiety to depression. Back in the forest . . . if you heard a twig snap it would not help your survival chances to dismiss it as 'probably a rabbit', so you conclude that it is probably a tiger—a huge tiger, and coming for you! Your brain is trying to spot the

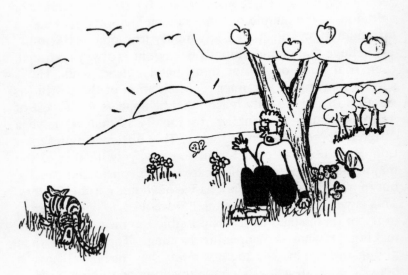

*Someone in a stressed state can be blinkered to everything but problems.*

tigers before they spot you, so it will err on the side of caution. You will have an image in your mind of a huge predator and, because we react physically and emotionally to what is playing in our minds, off goes the fight-or-flight response again even though nothing is actually there. *We call this worrying.* The world becomes a threatening place and confidence is lost.

If you were in a forest full of tigers (and as far as the fight-or-flight response is concerned *any* problem is a potential tiger), you would not stop for a nap—it would not help your survival. Of course, you might fall asleep exhausted but, as soon as the initial exhaustion had been slept off, you would wake very suddenly—totally alert and looking for tigers. You may have experienced this phenomenon yourself, or found it happening with patients: you fall asleep at night but wake suddenly around 2 a.m. and instantly start worrying about your own particular 'tigers'.

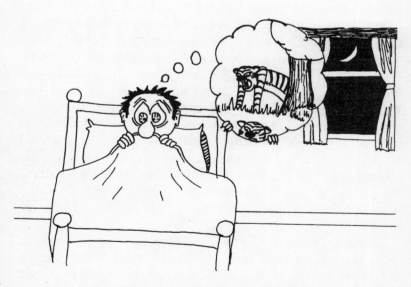

*. . . waking in the night and worrying about 'tigers' . . .*

In that same forest, full of potential tigers, it would be no kind of a survival trait to stop and smell the hibiscus, read something distracting or admire the sunset glinting through the lianas—that way, you could get eaten. Have you ever found yourself reading a paragraph of a book, and realising that none of it has sunk in? Then you go back and read it again with your lips moving, as if, miraculously, this will make it go in. People suffering from stress often find their powers of concentration failing. They may also lose interest in hobbies or other things they formerly enjoyed, often losing their sense of humour as well. In addition, the urge to procreate is subdued by the urge to survive (after all, it would not be a survival trait, during flight from the tiger, to become distracted by someone of the opposite sex), so impotence and frigidity can occur, denying opportunities for sexual release and physical comfort.

Patients often appear wrapped up in their own problems and fail to 'count their blessings'. Sometimes they say to me, 'I know I have a lot to be thankful for; there are lots of people worse off than me.' I am not a great advocate of the 'count your blessings' school of philosophy as a means of raising a patient's spirits, as it is this very survival instinct which, for very good reasons, makes people with problems focus on their own situation. Well-meaning friends and family who tell them to 'cheer up because there are lots worse off' often only serve to make patients feel guilty as well as frightened. Very often these (apparently) well-meaning people are really saying, 'I wish you would cheer up and be happy, because I don't know how to deal with your fear and misery.' But thinking of the starving in Africa, or of all the people who are more seriously ill than they are, often does not improve patients' prognosis or quality of life one jot.

However, there *are* ways of helping patients to focus on what is good in their lives, to modify their 'filters' as an aid to improving their well-being, and there are exercises designed precisely for this purpose later in the book (see

p. 149). If patients' stress *can* be reduced, one by-product, as they focus less on the 'tigers', will be an interest in things happening around them.

\* \* \*

In this chapter we have looked at what stress is—basically, it is anything we have to adapt to—how it affects people, and how it is often the way we are 'playing' reality that causes us stress. We react to this internal 'movie' as if it *were* reality. Later in the book we will explore ways of dealing with this 'reality', to help our patients cope with what is happening to them. Now, though, would be a good time to explain a procedure that makes good use of internal movies to help patients deal with tests and treatment. It is an adaptation of neuro-linguistic programming's 'new behaviour generator', and also very similar to the way sports psychologists prepare athletes for competition.

## MENTAL REHEARSAL

Because what we play in our internal 'cinema' is our reality, then anything that we have played over a few times becomes almost as familiar as if we had already experienced it; we do not have to adapt from scratch to the new situation, as it is not totally unfamiliar. Sports psychologists have their athletes mentally rehearsing, say, doing a high jump perfectly over and over again. Then when the big day arrives the routine is so familiar that the brain already has a 'groove' to run in—a habit formed—so the unconscious, rather than the conscious, mind can run the behaviour. Studies have shown that this can be a very effective way of rehearsing.

Typically, a patient who is due to have unfamiliar tests or treatments such as scans, biopsies, chemotherapy and radio-therapy will repeatedly imagine what is to come—the fight-

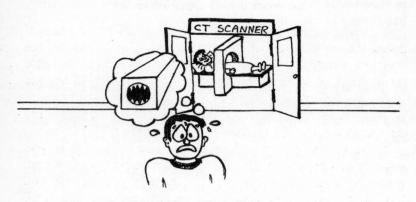

*Explaining the scanner will bring his anxiety down.*

or-flight response ensures that the threats become magnified—and his fear mounts. One way of reducing this fear is to introduce him in advance to the people and equipment he will encounter. Often simply explaining that the CT scanner is not a long dark tunnel, but more like a hoop, will bring stress down dramatically, particularly in a claustrophobic person. For some reason, pictures of CT scanners are only ever taken from the front, apparently showing the patient disappearing head first into a narrow tube. I explain to patients that the probable reason for photographs being taken this way, from the front, is because the front is all there is—like a stage set. The scanner is like a wall with a hole in it and the patient passes through it, not *into* it; I usually draw a couple of diagrams if I cannot show them the actual machine.

Once you have prepared your patient by providing him with the information he needs to familiarise himself with the procedure to come, you can teach him the following simple routine so that, when it is actually upon him, he will find it much easier to remain calm and comfortable.

### *The mental rehearsal exercise*

1    Imagine that you are about to direct a film of yourself
going through the test, the treatment and so on in exactly the
way you would *like* to deal with it—relaxed and comfortable
throughout. You are in the director's chair and watching the
'cast', including your stand-in, play the scene to your satisfaction. It is not important that you do not have all the
details of what will happen—just your version of it is fine.

2    Have the cast run through the scene exactly as you
want it to happen—with your stand-in remaining relaxed,
breathing easily and being perfectly comfortable. (If you
have been practising relaxation techniques you can have
your stand-in practising them as part of the scene.) Watch
all the other characters—doctors, nurses and technicians—
remaining relaxed because 'you' are relaxed and at ease.

3    When you have got the scene exactly as you would
like it, leave the director's chair, dismiss your stand-in, and
step into your role. Go through the scene again, playing
your part exactly as you had your stand-in do it—feeling
yourself relaxing and remaining comfortable throughout the
procedure.

4    If you are content with how it has gone, all you
have to decide is what will be your 'trigger' to begin
this—what will become automatic—behaviour. When will it
be most useful to have this behaviour start? What would
be a good signal to let your brain know to begin this
new habit? Will it be immediately you go through the
door of the room where it will happen? Or, maybe, when
you get on to the machine or sit in the chair for treatment? It could be when the porter arrives to take you to
the particular department. Decide on something that you
will see, hear, feel, smell or taste that you would like to
be the 'switch' to begin your new remaining-relaxed-and-
comfortable behaviour. Then go through your 'movie'
again, making sure that your chosen 'switch' is very clearly
included at the very beginning.

If you were *not* happy with the way your movie went, step back out and redirect it until you *are* happy with it.

When you have honed it to your satisfaction, all you have to do, whenever you have a few moments, is to close your eyes and go through it (playing your own part), making sure to include your 'switch'. By the time you actually have the tests or treatment the situation will seem very familiar to you, and your brain will automatically begin to go into the routine you have practised.

So, stress increases anxiety and anxiety increases stress. Stress causes problems with eating and sleeping; problems associated with energy, pain and emotional well-being. These problems then become stressors, and the symptoms spiral. It seems to me self-evident that, by reducing stress at every possible opportunity, we can improve the quality of life of our patients and their carers enormously, help them to deal with the symptoms of their disease and to get the best possible results from their treatment.

# 2   Good Communication

I believe that stress reduction is not something that should be exclusively reserved for particular sessions—it should be part of our every dealing with a patient (and his carers). If, every time you communicate with a person, you can leave him feeling more relaxed, listened to and understood, then you will go a long way towards improving his lot. **Gaining rapport** with a patient will make him feel more secure and much less stressed; it is also the way to gain empathy. It is worth remembering that to gain rapport with another person it is not necessary to like him or her. We all come across patients that we do not find particularly likeable—the patient population, just like the rest of the world, is made up of a cross-section of personalities. In my experience people do not turn into saints the moment they receive a diagnosis of cancer; indeed, someone under severe stress often appears selfish and bad-tempered. Gaining rapport is a way of building bridges, of increasing trust and communication.

There are simple ways in which you can gain rapport quickly, easily and consistently; ways that need a little practice at first but which quickly become 'natural', so that you no longer even have to do them consciously. It is a strange phenomenon that we like people who we think are like us. If we perceive another person to be like us, then that person feels familiar and comfortable to be with, and one of the best ways of giving another person the impression that you are like him is to **mirror** him. Anything you can observe about him you can mirror, with certain exceptions which I will come to a little later.

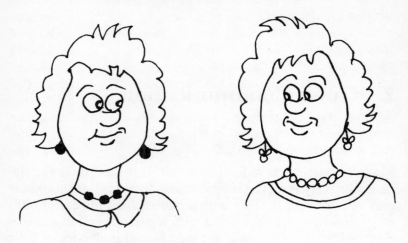

*We like people who we think are like us . . .*

## MIRRORING

You can mirror a person's posture. For instance, if he is sitting opposite you with his left leg crossed over his right at the knee, then you mirror him by crossing your right leg over your left (as in a mirror image)—it could be just at the ankle, because it does not need to be an exact copy. Similarly, if his arms are folded (contrary to popular body language theories this does not necessarily mean that he is putting up barriers—maybe it really is comfortable that way) you can fold your hands in your lap. If he is sitting forward in his chair, as is common in someone who is tense, then you too sit forward. When he changes posture, you simply change your posture to mirror his; and just as it does not have to be an exact copy, neither does it have to be immediate. (Bear in mind, though, that trying to be surreptitious can sometimes be very obvious.)

Do not worry that the other person will spot what you are doing! I was once asked to help coach a squad of disabled shooters with their concentration, motivation and confidence, and, since what I know about shooting can easily be written on a postcard, I set up a meeting with the person who was organising the coaching. After an hour and a half of discussing the topic and outlining a course of action, when I got up to leave I found that my right foot had 'gone to sleep', as I had been sitting on her sofa with my foot tucked under me. This is not a position I would normally adopt, as I am too large, but realisation dawned that the woman was an amputee—her left leg was missing from the knee. I had unconsciously mirrored her—and we had got on like the proverbial house on fire.

You can mirror another person's eye blink rate. Again, it does not have to be instant because it is the *rate* of blink you are mirroring. When someone is tense they often speak more quickly and pitch their voice higher; if you choose to mirror these features, make sure to keep your voice slightly slower and lower than the other person's, or you may make him feel even more tense.

The most powerful thing you can mirror is a person's breathing rate; after all, breathing is central to our existence. But there are certain guidelines to follow when mirroring breathing:

- *Do not* attempt to mirror breathing if your 'subject' is experiencing respiratory distress such as happens in hyperventilation, asthma, emphysema or COAD, as this will merely worsen the problem—and you are in danger of presenting an unprofessional image if you collapse.
- *Do not* stare at your patient's chest to discover her breathing rate—she will find this disconcerting and probably dismiss you as weird. You can still maintain eye contact but at the same time, with your peripheral vision, perceive her shoulders rising and falling or the pattern on her clothes moving. If the other person is speaking, it is a fair bet that she is breathing out (if you try to speak whilst inhaling you will discover that it is impossible), so you can begin to mirror the way she is breathing then.

As I said, breathing is one of the most powerful things you

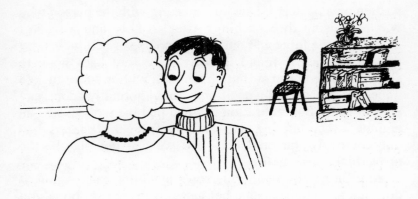

***Do not*** *stare at her chest.*

can mirror. So, if there are reasons why you cannot mirror the other person's breathing with your own, you can **cross-mirror**—that is, mirror his breathing with, say, slight hand or foot movements. He will take this in at an unconscious level.

It may be hard to believe that slight movements of the hand in response to your patient's breathing will be registered at *any* level, but we all take in far, far more information than we are consciously aware of. Have you ever encountered someone you know and immediately thought that he or she looked depressed? Was this piece of intuition arrived at with mystical powers? Telepathy, perhaps? No, something even more amazing happened. In a split second you noticed his skin tone was dull, his breathing was slow and low down in his abdomen, his shoulders slumped forwards, his gait was heavy and slow, and his eyes (if he is right-handed) were looking down and to his right. If he spoke at all it was probably slowly and in a flat voice. You did not have to go through a mental check-list, item by item: you observed all this unconsciously, then compared it with other examples in your memory bank of people displaying these features, and also with earlier examples of the person concerned. *Then* you immediately came to your educated guess that he was depressed—and all this you did in milliseconds. I used to think that I was very intuitive about people, until I 'got NLP' and realised that I was just good at reading their non-verbal signals. This may have come about from frequently having hearing problems as a child, when I had to make sense of the bits of language I was picking up by watching facial expressions and reading lips. If you wish to heighten your sensory awareness and therefore your 'intuition', try some of the exercises at the end of this chapter.

The 'subject' will take in unconsciously that you are mirroring, and the resulting feeling will be that you are comfortable and somehow familiar to be with. Of course you are—what he is seeing is himself! It is a standing joke amongst my friends that, during any gathering when I am in conversation with a stranger for more than a few seconds, he or she inevitably says something like, 'Don't I know you from somewhere? You seem familiar.' This is because I am a compulsive mirrorer.

As I said earlier, almost anything you can observe you can mirror. **But** I would warn against mirroring mannerisms that the other person is aware of, such as a nervous tic or a stammer! I have a habit of nodding and shaking my head at the same time, which I am aware of doing only when someone mentions it. I was once part of a group being 'taught' about a certain aspect of neuro-linguistic programming by someone who was managing to make an intriguing subject incomprehensible. He began answering my questions and, to my horror, nodding and shaking his head as he spoke. I was absolutely incensed that he should take the mickey in this way! Then I realised that my exasperation with his teaching must have shown in my face or voice and he, realising this, had begun to mirror me in an effort to regain rapport—unfortunately picking on the one thing guaranteed to wind me up!

Mirroring, then, is used to gain rapport, which is an extremely useful end in itself; but once you have rapport you can use it for even more benefit for your patient, by leading her into a relaxed and resourceful state. You can mirror whenever you communicate with your patient, even when taking details on admission ('What do you like to be called? Have you any pets at home?') when taking down her history.

### The mirroring exercise

1   Choose what you are going to mirror; you do not have to mirror *everything* that is happening—posture will do, but posture plus breathing will sometimes yield startling results.

2   Continue to mirror for a few minutes—this continuous mirroring is known as **pacing**.

You may feel that you could never get the hang of doing all this while still managing to hold a meaningful conversation. If you have ever learned to drive, do you remember the problems you had with three pedals and only two feet? As well as only two hands to control the direction of the car, and operate the indicators, wipers, horn, lights, gears and handbrake. Plus, the car was moving and there were other cars out there, also moving! Well the good news is that mirroring, pacing and leading (see 3 below) are much easier to learn than driving. Furthermore, errors are not usually fatal. Just as with any skill, though, you have to go through four stages:

i    unconscious incompetence—you do not know that you cannot do it, because you have not tried yet;

ii   conscious incompetence—you try it and find out you cannot do it;

iii  conscious competence—if you concentrate and try hard you can do it most of the time;

iv   unconscious competence—you can do it without even thinking about it. (You reach the point in driving when you get into the car, drive off while singing along to the radio or chatting to your passenger, eating an apple and looking in shop windows.)

Practise one or two aspects of mirroring until they become unconscious; then you can, if you wish, add more.

3   When you judge that you are getting on reasonably well, begin to change your own posture to a more relaxed position (this is called **leading**), very gradually. Observe the other person and, if you have rapport, she will begin to follow your movements. If this does not occur, simply continue to pace a little longer, then try again until it does happen. If it is breathing that you are mirroring, after a while begin to slow your own breathing while watching for her response. Apply the same techniques for eye blinks, pitch and tone of voice, or with cross-mirroring. Your patient will begin to feel 'better', more relaxed, understood and secure without even knowing why.

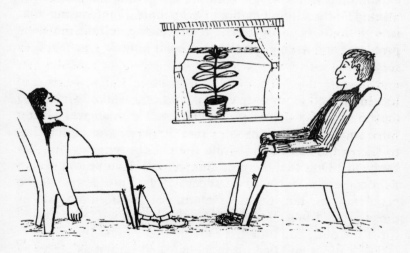

*If you have rapport, he will begin to follow your lead.*

These techniques were arrived at by observing people who are natural communicators: they unconsciously mirror other people. Watch couples in pubs and restaurants and notice which seem to be getting on really well together, then notice their posture.

4    There is one more thing to add in regard to mirroring, pacing and leading. When you need to break off to do something else—when the communication is at an end for that occasion—then you need to break the link temporarily. You can do this in many ways, but whichever you choose you must do it decisively by **mismatching** whatever you were pacing. If you fail to do this it will not have terrible consequences, but you may have difficulty in getting on with the rest of your life! I taught these techniques to a research staff member at one of my hospitals but neglected to tell her about mismatching. She accosted me in the corridor and said, 'I'm having problems with this mirroring stuff.' I was perplexed, as I am always very pleased with the results of these techniques, so I asked her if I had not explained it well enough—wasn't she getting the results she wanted? She said, 'Oh no, it's brilliant. I'm finding that new patients open up to me really easily, telling me their problems and asking questions . . . but *how do I get them to shut up*?'

I once arrived at an outpatients' unit and walked right into the middle of a drama. A middle-aged woman was sitting there sobbing, almost hysterically. Someone was attempting to take a blood sample, while the patient was begging her husband, 'Don't let them do this to me!' A nurse was trying to console her, but with no success. I had no idea what the problem was, but it was escalating at an alarming rate as those around her attempted to calm her down. So I called for 'time out', and took her into another room.

The patient huddled up in a chair and turned as far away from me as was physically possible—I was obviously 'one of them', and she was having nothing to do with me. She flatly refused to speak to me, and it was left to her harassed husband to tell me what was happening. He was upset, but also furious, as she was refusing chemotherapy because she had just been told that she would lose her hair. He just could not understand why she would risk her life for something (to him) so trivial. This news had in fact been the last straw in a long saga of problems, and she was adamant that she would not have the treatment.

Because she was still refusing to acknowledge me and staring resolutely out of the window, from time to time sobbing, I continued to talk to her husband but began to mirror her. I cross-mirrored her breathing with my hand resting on my chair arm, as I knew it would be within her peripheral vision, and also with my voice, pacing my sentences to her exhalations. This was not completely perfect, but it does not have to be.

During my discussion with her husband I also began to pace her experience; anyone familiar with counselling will already (hopefully) be used to working like this. In this case it took the form of my agreeing with her—via my conversation with her husband—that losing your hair *is* extremely upsetting, especially to someone who obviously takes pride in her appearance, and so on. If I had agreed with her husband that 'losing your hair for a few months is a small price to pay for your life', I would probably never have gained rapport. After a few minutes of this she turned round and hurled abuse at him for not supporting her but, after I had 'refereed' for a little while, she realised that she and her husband were both on the same side. I continued to mirror, pace and lead until I managed to help her sit back in the armchair in a more relaxed position, and we were able to discuss her difficulties and how best *we* might deal with them.

For the first week or two I phoned her regularly and continued to mirror, pace and lead, using voice and breathing, and pacing her experience of the situation. She got herself organised with a designer wig, worked out coping strategies and, after this traumatic start, sailed through the treatment. She is now more than happy to talk to other patients facing the same ordeal, and often laughs about how rude she was to me.

I find it really difficult to quote specific case histories to support these methods, simply because I use them whenever I am dealing with another person. My metaphor for mirroring, pacing and leading—and for rapport—is that of radio waves carrying transmissions from one point to another. You hear the words on your radio, not the radio waves. But, without the radio waves, the words would never reach their audience. I believe that rapport and non-verbal signals are essential to effective communication between individuals. It has been estimated that words contribute only around 7 per cent of the impact of communication between people; tone of voice, approximately 38 per cent; and body language (posture, gestures and eye contact) determines the remaining 55 per cent.

POINTS TO REMEMBER ABOUT MIRRORING
*Do not*
*mimic*; that is, do not attempt to do exactly what the other person is doing at the precise moment she is doing it. If she twiddles her ring, wait a moment and adjust your watch strap; if she runs her hand through her hair, you could rub your earlobe. If you mimic, she will register that something is amiss.
*mirror mannerisms or nervous gestures.*
*Peer at the part of her that you are mirroring*—use your peripheral vision.

*Do*
*cross-mirror if your patient has respiratory problems*—use small hand or foot movements instead.
*pace her experience, her reality*—as with the young woman mentioned (on p. 35), it is important to validate her concerns rather than brush them aside. *Then* you can hopefully lead her to a more resourceful state.

Before leaving this topic I would like to include a very simple technique that is useful, where other methods of communication may be ineffectual, in calming someone who is confused and agitated. Sit beside the patient's bed or chair and rest your hand on his forearm—a very natural thing to do—but hold the arm a little more firmly than you normally would. In essence, you are mirroring his own muscle tension because, if your patient is tense or agitated, it is unlikely that he will have relaxed muscles. As with other methods of mirroring, pacing and leading, pace for a little while, then begin to lead by very gradually releasing your grip. Notice if the person begins to relax and, if he does, continue to relax your own hand. If not, continue to pace a little longer, then try again. This technique is doubly effective if you can also mirror (or cross-mirror) breathing at the same time).

## THE POWER OF LANGUAGE

As I said earlier, pacing language is extremely important if you are to gain rapport with a patient. A person's choice of words is how he illustrates his reality to the outside world— and we all have different realities. We can never know how another person is feeling—even if we have had similar experiences—because we are not him and we have a different set of 'filters'. We can only ever hope to get close to understanding what he is experiencing, and the closer we can get then the more rapport and empathy we will have. I would hope that any competent health care professional would choose her words according to the person with whom she is communicating. You probably would not make an elderly, timid and refined lady feel understood and secure if you used the same approach as you would with a thirty-year-old labourer with a history of alcohol or drug abuse and grievous bodily harm (or vice versa!). There are different and subtle ways of using language to communicate well with different patients.

We tend to believe that everyone else thinks in the same way that we think, but if you listen carefully to a person's language you will begin to notice that he probably fits into one of the following categories:

1   *visual thinkers*, who think mainly in pictures (we all do
    this to some degree). These people appear to think
    quickly, are usually good spellers and can become un-
    comfortable in surroundings that are cluttered or un-
    pleasant to the eye. Their language illustrates that they
    are mainly visual, as they tend to use expressions like:
      I can *see* what you mean.
      There's no *light* at the end of the tunnel.
      *See* if you can *shed some light* on the situation.
      He *brightens* my life.
      Her language is certainly *colourful*!
2   *auditory thinkers*, who hold mental conversations with
    themselves, have internal discussions with themselves
    before acting. They appear to think and read more
    slowly than visuals because they think and read at the
    speed of the spoken word. They can become uncomfort-
    able if there are loud or discordant noises around them
    (it drowns out their internal dialogue). You will often
    hear them use expressions like:
      It *sounds* reasonable to me.
      That has the *ring* of truth to it.
      You've *pitched* that about right.
      I'd like a little peace and *harmony*!
3   *kinesthetic* (feeling) *thinkers*, who have 'intuitions' and
    'gut feelings' and go with what feels right. To feel
    relaxed they need their clothing, temperature and fur-
    nishings to be comfortable. If you listen you may catch
    them using expressions like:
      I feel *crushed* by what's happened.
      It's too much to *bear*.
      I just can't get a *handle* on what's happening to me.

  We are all a mixture of these three categories, as well as
having features of another, called

4   *digital thinkers*, who use precise language which con-
    tains few of the types of phrases mentioned in categories
    1 to 3; it is almost 'computer-speak'. These people often

appear logical and analytical. Party political broadcasts are often written in this manner; they use expressions such as:

I completely understand.

That is proving to be difficult.

I cannot comprehend how that happened.

Do you think you could do that?

Notice how these last sentences contain no visual, auditory or kinesthetic language. As I said, we are all a mixture of these types, but most people have a preferred system and use the language that suits their way of thinking. If you really want to use the subtleties of language to help your rapport, then spend a little time polishing up your awareness of the different types of language that people use— while watching chat shows on TV, for example. Or, during telephone conversations, keep a notepad handy and put column headings of V, A, K and D (optional). Each time you spot or hear a word or phrase from one of the categories put a tick in the appropriate column. You will soon find out if the person you are listening to has a preferred system.

Once you have polished up your awareness, you can start using your patients' own language systems. For instance, if a patient said, 'My nerves are just jangling, I could scream!', and you replied with 'Yes, I can see you're having a problem', then she would be likely to think that you were not hearing what she was saying! She described to you exactly what was happening in her head—what she was hearing inside; you replied by telling her that you could *see* what she was hearing! If you had replied with something like, 'It sounds to me as if we need to find a way of bringing a little peace and harmony into your life,' she would have immediately felt that you understood exactly what was needed.

If a patient confided, 'I can't bear this any more. I just feel that I'm carrying the weight of the world on my shoulders', he would obviously be using kinesthetic (feeling) language.

You would increase your rapport and help him to feel that you grasped what he meant by replying, for instance, 'We will try to give you the support you need to lighten the load.' This is more likely to help him feel understood than, 'It must appear that there is no light at the end of the tunnel.'

These are not meant to be 'scripts' to be used verbatim, of course—they are just my attempt to illustrate further ways that will help your patients to feel that you understand a little more of their reality.

*The power of words cannot be overestimated* in our dealings with patients. Just as they let us know what is happening in their heads by the language they use, so too the words we choose can have an effect on their internal processes. You have probably heard it said that people illustrate their attitude to life by whether they describe a glass as being 'half empty' or 'half full'. They are describing the same object, but making a different meaning from it. I have often been witness to a similar phenomenon during medicine rounds on the wards—when, for instance, a group of male patients are watching football on someone's TV. The atmosphere is jovial and relaxed as they are all absorbed in the game. Then along comes the drugs trolley and the nurse says something like, 'Anyone need anything for pain?' From being externally focused on the football and each other, they are suddenly jolted into focusing on themselves and scanning for pain. Suddenly their shoulders slump and their skin tone alters and their jovial conversation falters.

Going back to what I said in Chapter 1 about filtering our experience—if you encourage a person to pass reality through a 'pain filter' then it is likely that he will find some, although until that moment he had been pleasantly distracted and comfortable. Even if he is not currently experiencing pain, he will consider whether he is likely to have any in the near future, remembering how unpleasant it is to suffer pain . . . so should he have something in case? If, on the other hand, the nurse on her drugs round had said, 'Everyone comfortable?' her words would have installed a 'comfort filter' through which to check the men's present state. Reality is what we focus on.

Often just paying a little attention to the tense we use when we are speaking to a patient can have an effect on her representation of reality. Read the following two sentences while trying to put yourself in the position of a frightened patient who has been having pain. Take a little time to notice how your internal representation is different for each one:

'Oh dear, you're having some pain?'
    Now try this one:
'Oh dear, you have had some pain?'

The first, in the present tense, helps the patient to get stuck in a painful 'now'; while the second sentence helps her to move forward by putting the pain in her past—if only temporarily. Patients often do get stuck, and it can help them enormously if you use language to get them moving again.

I frequently see patients who have had successful surgery for breast cancer, with no evidence of remaining disease, and who are about to have radiotherapy and chemotherapy as a back-up. For them it is easy to become stuck in the horror of the diagnosis, to regard themselves as cancer sufferers, even though their current state of health is good. This, of course, is partly due to the fact that they are still attending for cancer treatment, even though this is now frequently given just as a preventive. With patients such as these, my object is to help them to move their sights to the future and to get on with their lives, rather than focusing on the recent past. With this always at the back of my mind, I liberally use the past tense when speaking with them— 'when you had cancer', or 'when you were ill', or perhaps 'when you look back to the time when you had cancer'. If a patient will be continuing with chemotherapy for a while, and those few months appear to stretch interminably before him, I often use questions such as, 'Six months from now—when you are looking back—what is it like?' To answer my question she has to mentally project herself six months into the future in order to imagine how it feels to have the surgery and treatment behind her.

Both my patients and I know the facts: that there is always a possibility of relapse; and, obviously, they need time to come to terms with what has happened to them. This can often be most fruitfully done when they have been able to put a little distance between themselves and their traumatic time. Usually the reason why patients allow themselves to be put through tests, surgery and follow-up treatment is to increase their chances of staying alive—and by this I mean *living*, not just functioning or existing. If they remain frozen to the spot like rabbits in car headlights, unable to move on, then they are not living, even though they are not dead. Language can be a powerful lever in helping them to begin moving forwards and regaining control again.

## HEIGHTEN YOUR SENSORY ACUITY

### *The cleansing-the-gates-of-perception exercise*

Essentially, this is an exercise that helps you to learn to look at things actively, dynamically and alertly. Usually when we look at something we think in words—'green', 'sharp', 'small' and so on. Or we tend to compare it with something similar that we have seen. The exercise I am about to describe is about *simply looking*; 'feeling' an object with the eyes, without mentally describing it. Close your eyes for a moment and stroke whatever material is covering your thigh; focus all your attention on how it feels to your hand, without putting it into words. You are about to do the equivalent with your eyes.

It is a difficult but rewarding exercise, which disciplines

the mind but also 'cleanses the gates of perception', heightening your powers of observation. This leads to an increased awareness of tiny changes in people (non-verbal communication), with resulting improvements in your rapport with them and your 'intuition' or ability to read them. Another benefit is that the world around you becomes richer, more colourful and diverse. Although it is intended here to enhance your communication skills with patients, it is also another technique in your repertoire that some of your patients could usefully learn from you. This is how you do it:

1    Choose a simple object—a pebble, twig or pine cone is fine (I learned to do this using a matchstick). Hold it a comfortable distance from your eyes and move it around as you look at it from different angles. Vary the distance from your eyes as you do this, or they will begin to ache, and just *look* without mentally describing ('That bit looks sharp') or comparing ('It's almost the colour of my kitchen ceiling'). It is almost as if you are stroking it with your eyes . . . just looking . . . and looking.

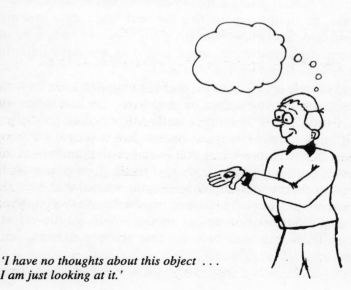

*'I have no thoughts about this object . . .*
*I am just looking at it.'*

Because you are using something fairly plain you will initially find this exercise pretty boring; but after a few short sessions of 5–10 minutes you will begin to notice tiny details, colours and textures that you previously missed, and at each session you will discover more. If you did this exercise with a complicated or multi-coloured object you would probably never develop your ability to see the minute details. I graduated from a matchstick to a small pine cone, and you would be amazed at the variety of colours and textures there were to be discovered!

2   Be kind to yourself, as it is very easy to become distracted and bored at first, until you begin to heighten your powers of observation. So gently bring your attention back each time you wander.

Just a few minutes daily can really make a difference to your skills in reading your patients' non-verbal communication (remember: posture, gestures and eye contact make up 55 per cent of communication!). If you wish to polish up your awareness of changes in their voices and, less obviously, their breathing, you could do a similar exercise involving listening to a simple piece of music. Avoid singing along mentally, anticipating the next few bars or making comparisons. Just close your eyes and listen to each note in turn, and each instrument, regarding it as a series of single notes or chords rather than a tune.

It takes only a few minutes daily to heighten your powers of observation—you do not have to lose your hearing to do it, as I did! You will be pleasantly surprised at how your 'intuition' improves as you discern tiny changes in your patients. Those times when you have felt that an individual was keeping something from you, that all was not as it seemed, were probably times when you noticed that what he was saying conflicted in some way with what you were receiving from his non-verbal signals. With a little effort, your skill in this area will become more consistent and reliable.

*      *      *

The following neuro-linguistic programming exercises, which are done in groups of four or five people, develop some of your other senses—some that might seem relatively unimportant. However, we use them all unconsciously, and it is *the total of all the information* that comes through all our channels that is processed before we make any meaning of a communication.

### NLP exercise 1

1 One group member, A, sits on a chair with her eyes closed.

2 The other members approach from the rear, one at a time, and rest one hand on the seated person's shoulder while announcing their names: 'This is Clare', and so on. When one moves away, the next group member carries out the same procedure (on the same shoulder each time), and this continues until everyone has announced who they are while resting one hand on the seated person's shoulder.

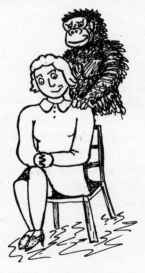

*Who can it be?*

3   The routine is carried out once more, in the same order.

4   In random order, each person in turn again approaches A and rests his hand on her shoulder, but without announcing who he is this time, and it is up to A to try to identify who is touching her shoulder, simply by how the hand feels (warmth, pressure, size and so forth).

5   If A guesses correctly, then the next person approaches silently and touches her shoulder. If the guess is incorrect, the person announces his name in order to allow A to 're-calibrate'; then the next person approaches.

6   This continues until A has scored a clear round, by successfully identifying each group member in turn. Then A rejoins the group and B takes the chair. This is repeated until all group members have had a clear round.

*Variation 1*
Repeat the above exercise, but with each person resting three fingers on the seated person's shoulder. Then, if you really want to refine your skills, try it with two fingers—then one!

*Variation 2*
Repeat the routine but this time each person, instead of placing his hand on A's shoulder, holds the palm of his hand in front of her nose while announcing his name. A takes a good long sniff, and the next person approaches. The exercise continues until everyone has had a clear round.

This exercise, and variations 1 and 2, each appear to rely on using a single sense, but unconsciously, while concentrating on smells, you will also be noticing things like radiated body warmth and breathing. Or when concentrating on touch, you will still be unconsciously registering scents and breathing, as well as the height from which the voice is coming. This particular variation is pretty subtle and may even seem vague, but it illustrates very effectively how much information we apparently gather from thin air.

*Variation 3*
Place another chair beside A's. In turn, as before, each member of the group announces his name, then sits in the chair for a few seconds. He then gets up and rejoins the group, and the next person repeats the routine. The exercise proceeds as before, until everyone has scored a clear round.

### NLP exercise 2

Now that you are beginning to enhance your sensory acuity, this exercise and its variations will help you to use these skills to read non-verbal signals. These 'games' require only yourself and one other person. Here are the steps:

1 Ask your partner to think about someone she really likes, without speaking to you. Notice her skin tone . . . are there any patches of high colour on her face? Notice the size of her lower lip . . . the shape of her mouth . . . and her eyes . . . How wide are her nostrils? What is her rate of

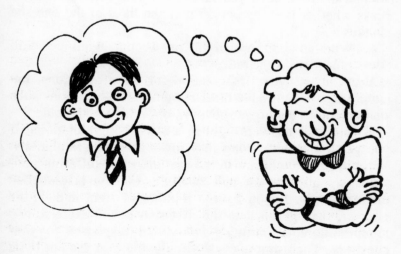

*Ask her to think about someone she really likes.*

respiration, and at what level is she breathing (high, middle or low)? Be aware of her posture . . . how is she holding her shoulders . . . and head?

2   When you think that you have had enough time to mentally note her non-verbal signals, ask her to think about something neutral (such as her 2 times table) for a few seconds.

3   Ask her to think about someone she dislikes, and again notice all her non-verbal communications and make mental notes.

If by now you are not reasonably confident that you noticed enough differences between the two sets of signals to tell them apart, repeat the procedure.

4   Now ask your partner, 'Which of these two people lives closer to you?' and, after giving her a couple of seconds to answer the question mentally, tell her—and base your judgement on her 'non-verbals'—whether she is thinking of the person she likes or the one she dislikes. Then she can tell you if you are right or wrong.

5   Whatever the answer, ask her the next question: 'Which of them have you known the longest?', and again guess whether it is the person that she likes or the one she dislikes.

6   Whether you are right or wrong, continue with 'Which of them is the tallest?'

You can use your imagination for other questions, but make sure they all have clear-cut answers—questions such as 'Which has the bigger house?', or 'Which is the older?'

If you get 4 answers right in a row—congratulations! If you get 4 answers wrong in a row—also congratulations! You have definitely registered that there are differing non-verbal signals for 'like' and 'dislike'; you have just labelled them wrongly. If you have a mixture of right and wrong guesses, then go back to the first step in the exercise and re-calibrate your partner's non-verbal responses to your questions. Then simply cycle through the exercise until you consistently guess right.

*Variation 1*

Ask your partner to think of someone he likes and, while doing this, to count aloud from 1 to 10 while you listen with your eyes closed; then to think of someone that he dislikes and, again, to count from 1 to 10 aloud. Have him do this until you are reasonably confident that you can tell the difference in his voice when he is talking about the one and when he is talking about the other. Now, ask him questions similar to those from the previous exercise, but this time he has to count aloud from 1 to 10 while thinking about the answer. The rest of this variation proceeds exactly as the previous one.

*Variation 2*

Sitting facing your partner, ask him a series of questions to which you already know the answer—and he has to answer in the affirmative even if his answer is untrue. It will go something like this: 'Is your name Fred?' (knowing that his name is actually Brian), and he has to answer, 'Yes, it is.' Notice his non-verbals as he lies to you.

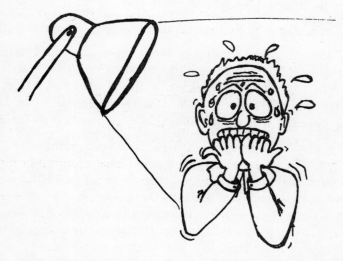

*You may find you can spot his non-verbals without too much difficulty.*

Ask a mixture of questions that will cause him sometimes to answer truthfully and at other times to lie, as he always has to answer with 'Yes/ I am/ I do/ I have' and so on. You can ask things like, 'Are you English/ Married/ an airline pilot/ a vegetarian?'

When you are satisfied that you can spot the differences in his non-verbal signals between when he is telling the truth and when he is lying, go on to ask questions to which you do *not* know the answers. In the interests of maintaining harmonious relations it is wise to stick to non-personal topics such as, 'Do you have double glazing/ like driving/ have gas central heating/ like Indian food/ enjoy flying?' He again replies in the affirmative to all your questions, and your task is to 'guess' whether he is telling the truth or not. Your partner tells you each time whether you have guessed correctly. When you have achieved 6 correct guesses in a row you can change places. Again, if you are consistently wrong, then you are aware of the differences in the other person's signals but you have labelled them wrongly. If your guesses are inconsistent, you need to ask him a few more preliminary questions until you are more sure of the differences.

As I said at the beginning of this chapter, I do not believe that stress management should be something reserved for discrete sessions. By making a little time and effort to master the skills that I have described here you can help your patients feel more secure, understood, cared-for and relaxed *every time* you have contact with them.

# 3  Living in the Now

Until this point I have concentrated on practical things to do with patients, but because I believe strongly in helping patients regain control of their well-being, this chapter is devoted to skills that you can teach to patients. Most of the techniques that I have covered so far have been taken or adapted from neuro-linguistic programming. I love NLP for its speed, its consistency, its respect for my patients' integrity and for its logic. Much of my joy in life and work derives from my 'having NLP' and from the tools it gives me. So it may seem a little strange that I am now going to devote a chapter to the apparently mystical subject of meditation.

Before going any further I must explain what meditation is *not*: meditation is not 'mind-blanking'. I do not know how to make my mind go blank; and if I did succeed in making my mind go blank, how would I know that I had done it? And how would I know when to stop doing it? Given that you have something as amazingly powerful as your mind, why would you want to turn it off when you could be learning how to use it to your best advantage?

I had the pleasure and privilege of studying meditation with Dr Lawrence Le Shan, an American psychologist and one of the founding fathers of the holistic approach to cancer. My studying meditation had to do with a belief that my reason for being on earth (if there *is* a reason) is to find out what it means to be fully human: what am I, and therefore other people too, capable of? As I said, meditation sounds pretty mystical after the preceding chapters! But not only did I find in it a route to discovering my humanhood—

I also discovered what a marvellous stress-proofer meditation is. There are countless ways of meditating, and for as
many different reasons, but I would like to concentrate on
meditation as **an antidote to stress** and as **a way of
improving quality of life**. What many methods have in
common is that they are about attempting to focus your
mind on one thing. I say 'attempt' because it is only when
you *try* to focus your mind on one thing that you realise
how difficult this task is!

Stop and think about stress/tension/anxiety/worry for a
moment . . . Much of it comes from thinking about things
that have (or have not) happened in the past; or from imagining what may (or, even more bizarre, may not) happen in the
future. As I explained in Chapter 1, the body reacts to what is
playing in the mind, so remembered and imagined events can
cause as much stress as current events.

## LIVING FULLY, IN THE PRESENT

If you can learn to focus on 'now' most of the time,
then you automatically reduce the stress from imagined or
remembered events. There are many studies on the benefits
of meditation—some claim that illness (as measured by
days in hospital or certified sickness benefit claims) is
halved in people who meditate. Ainslie Meares, a distin-
guished Australian psychiatrist, developed what he called
'ataraxis'—a form of meditation—and wrote of its benefits
for people dealing with cancer. Whatever you believe about
the claims for meditation, its physiological stress-proofing
effects are difficult to disprove, with all the implications for
pain, breathing, sleeping, eating and anxiety.

There *are* many different types of meditation, for all
manner of purposes, but they all tend to offer the same
beneficial physical and emotional benefits—the opposite of
the fight-or-flight response. There are certain indicators for
measuring these benefits, such as a lowered metabolic rate
and subsequent reducing of oxygen consumption; reduction

in heartbeat; and a sharp decrease in blood lactate levels (this happens almost four times faster during meditation than in someone resting quietly in a safe place; blood lactate level is one indicator of anxiety and tension levels). Add to this the personality-strengthening effects, and you can begin to see why I am such a keen advocate of meditation!

Of course, not all patients are willing or able to learn how to meditate. It requires self-discipline and a desire to take some responsibility for one's own well-being. For those who do choose to try it, the benefits repay their efforts. I have noticed that those patients who practise self-help techniques such as relaxation and meditation tend to live better, if not longer. It often seems to happen that such patients live for the predicted length of time, but remain comparatively well for most of it, with just a short decline at the end. A good quality of life does appear to be maintained for longer.

If you believe that meditation is 'airy-fairy' and that it is only for saffron-robed vegetarians, or for hippies sitting cross-legged and chanting 'Ohm . . .', then what follows will be fairly boring! Meditation is a mind discipline that often depends on the repeated practice of boring tasks. People who do press-ups do so for the long-term benefits of increased stamina and muscle strength, and that is the way it is with meditation. Intrinsically it is pointless and potentially boring, but the pay-off is increased powers of concentration and memory, reduced stress (with all its implications) and a much greater ability to live **in the now**, to focus on what you wish to focus on. And what you focus on *is* your reality (remember the red Fiestas in Chapter 1?)

We would all, at times, benefit from living more fully in the now—more so if our future had been curtailed because of a poor prognosis. Many of the good times, the happy/funny/satisfying times, are wasted by thinking about the past and the possible future. We have a habit of remembering the 'good old days'; unfortunately, we often miss

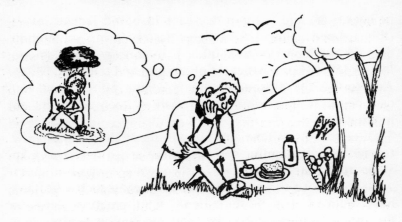

*Living in the now can be a lot more rewarding.*

them while they are actually happening because we are too busy remembering earlier 'good old days' or worrying about what might be to come. Whatever our state of health or our prognosis, we can improve our quality of life if we choose what we are focusing our attention on rather than letting our minds run disaster movies as if we have no choice in what we think about. Meditation can help us choose the 'movie' that is playing in our head. Later in the book come more ways of changing and redirecting the movies—of realising that we *are* the director and projectionist of our imagination. But for now . . .

### The breath-counting meditation

This is not a physical relaxation exercise; it is meant to be done in an alert manner (remember, this is mental press-ups), and the stress-reducing benefits come from controlling the mind. If the mind is calm, then the physical benefits will follow.

The 'rules' for this one are really simple: you just have to mentally count your exhalations in 4s. That is, when breathing out you mentally count the breaths until you reach 4, then start again. It is marginally easier if you mentally add an 'and' on the inhalation. I say 'marginally' because the idea is to try to think of nothing else but counting your breaths, and it is impossible to actually do! You will find your mind wandering off in all sorts of directions . . . and this may be the first time that you discover that your mind has a mind of its own!

For this meditation, encourage your patients to sit up if possible, or at least to avoid a sleeping position. Of course, this type of meditation is unsuitable for patients with respiratory problems; but you could teach them one of the other meditation methods in this chapter. It is difficult to remain alert enough to practise this technique after a heavy meal or when really tired, so have them avoid these times. Remember, the idea is not for them to drift into sleep, but to learn to focus their minds. Having said that, it is slightly easier if they close their eyes to avoid outside distractions.

Patients may find that they begin thinking about what they are going to have for lunch; or that their nose is itching (in which case, scratch it!); that this is a damned boring meditation (which it is, initially); or even how well they are doing. Lawrence Le Shan calls this 'the law of the good moment' or 'here I am, wasn't I?', because when you realise how well you are doing you have just 'shot yourself in the foot'—you are supposed to be thinking *only* about counting your breaths!

The mind struggles against this enforced discipline and will probably try to distract by making mental pictures of the numbers—seeing them on doors, blackboards, dials and so on. If this happens it's fine—as long as you stay with the first representation of numbers that appears—this is important for the discipline. If the numbers change appearance, then the idea is to gently, but firmly, change them back; you can always use the new format next time!

It will help you to understand this meditation, before you teach it to patients, if you try it out yourself for a while. You have nothing to lose but stress, anxiety, insomnia, muscle tension, so:

1   Sit upright in an alert manner; close your eyes and begin to notice the rhythm of your breathing.

2   Begin to count your exhalations, with an 'and' on each inhalation: 'And . . . one . . . and . . . two . . . and . . . three . . . and . . . four . . . and . . . one . . .'

3   When you find yourself being distracted by thoughts or images or external stimuli, brush them gently aside (being very kind to yourself because this *is* an impossible task) and go back to the job in hand, which is simply(?) thinking about nothing else but counting your exhalations.

4   When you have finished your meditation session open your eyes and sit quietly for a couple of minutes to allow your mind and body (which will have slowed down) to readjust before doing anything else.

This meditation is a little like training a lively and curious puppy to walk at heel. You have it on the lead and set out for a walk to the shops, but it has ideas of its own. It constantly strains at the lead, dashing off to one side to sniff at another dog, then to a tree on the other side. It gets under your feet and trips you up, and crossing roads becomes a risky business. Gradually, though, you begin to train it by gently tugging the lead when the puppy strays off. This way you reach your destination much more easily. You can even take your dog to the park and let it off the lead to roam and run freely, knowing that you have trained it to return when you call.

As I have already warned you, initially this meditation can be incredibly boring. But this is part of the discipline, and after a few sessions you begin to feel calmed and centred; that you are 'the right person in the right place at the right time'. It is easiest to begin with a five-minute session daily, increasing this to a fifteen- or twenty-minute session daily over a week or so. It is OK to glance at a clock or watch to check your progress; but do not set an alarm, or

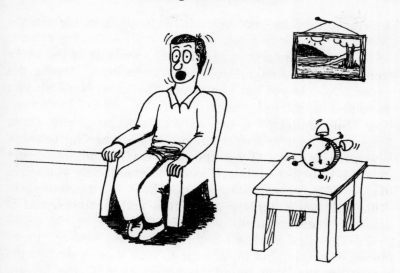

*Do **not** set an alarm.*

you will experience a sensation similar to being jolted from sleep by the phone or doorbell. Soon you will find that you can judge when your time is up, and you will also find that the time seems very brief.

### The mantra meditation

A mantra is simply a word, sound or phrase repeated, audibly or mentally, over and over again with the intention of focusing on nothing else but the word(s). Some schools of meditation insist, for various reasons, that the words be carefully chosen, but for the purposes of mental discipline, of learning to live in the now and of reducing stress it does not matter a great deal which words or sounds are chosen (as long as you steer clear of words with a negative content, like 'death' or 'pain'!).

It is probably easier to do a mantra meditation using a nonsense word that has no connotations whatsoever.

Lawrence Le Shan recommends his method for choosing a word: let the phone book fall open and, with eyes closed, stick your finger on the page. The first syllable of the name you hit is the first syllable of your mantra. Repeat the procedure, and you get your second syllable. Now, all you have to do is the following:

1   Sit comfortably, but without slouching, and chant your word over and over again while attempting to think about nothing else. If you choose to do it aloud, make sure that it is only just audible; if you chant too loudly you are in danger of hyperventilating as you take in too much oxygen. This will cause tingling extremities and dizziness, and is not to be recommended!

2   The idea is to do nothing but the chanting, to be aware of nothing but the chanting. Stick with it, despite the variations that your mind produces. As with the breath-counting meditation, you will probably find that your mind plays all kinds of tricks. It will try to make meaning from a nonsense word; it will begin to make puns or rhymes. Keep bringing your mind back to just concentrating on your chanting.

Try one mantra for five to eight sessions before you decide whether it is right for you; and if it *is* right, you will find yourself succeeding in just chanting for up to 20 seconds at a time. You can try nonsense mantras using the phone book or other method, or use specific words or phrases, depending on your preference. Some people prefer to use words such as 'calm', 'tranquil', 'peace' or 'heal'. It is very much a matter of 'suck it and see'.

Whatever mantra you choose, it is all about disciplining and calming the mind—about focusing on the now. As with all types of meditation, it should be practised every day for an increasing length of time, up to a maximum 30-minute daily session. After a month of one type, it should be obvious whether you are deriving any benefit.

## *The bubble meditation*

This is intended to help slow down the stream of consciousness and to help you to become detached from it. Although, strictly speaking, this too should be done in an alert manner, it can be a wonderful aid to sleeping if a patient is troubled by thoughts rushing through her mind (a common problem). Purists might criticise the use of this meditation to help a person drift off to sleep, but laying awake in the early hours worrying is not going to help anyone's daytime energy levels. As with many of the techniques in this book, I have adapted this one to the needs of people dealing with illness, and I feel the end justifies the means! If you teach this meditation to a patient, try to ensure that she reserves it *either* for alert daytime use *or* for sleeping.

There are three scenarios for doing the bubble meditation. Sticking to the chosen one is important for success, so your patient should pick the one that appeals the most (if necessary, after trying out all three a few times).

1   Imagine that you are sitting on the bottom of a deep, clear lake, waiting for thoughts to pop into your mind (as they inevitably will). Each time a thought enters your head, put it into a bubble: a large bubble, which rises to the surface of the lake taking 5–7 seconds to do so.

As your thought rises, simply observe it in a detached manner: 'That's what I am thinking now.' Do this almost as if you are observing someone else's thoughts, making no attempt to connect the thoughts or direct them. Whatever comes into your head is fine. It may be that the same thought keeps appearing for a while, and that's fine too; just keep observing, and it will eventually be replaced with another thought. You might think, 'I can't think of anything to think', but that is a thought too. As I explained in the previous chapter, we all have different ways of thinking: some of us in pictures, some in words and some in feelings. Well, however your thoughts appear, be it in pictures or in printed words, internal dialogue or just feelings, they can go slowly up to the surface in a bubble.

Then just sit and wait for the next thought to appear—making no effort to choose it, to make sense of it, or to get involved with it. Just observe it for those few seconds, then wait for the next one to come along. The idea is not to find any deep and meaningful insights or answers (though this may happen), but merely to control the speed at which the thoughts pass through your mind and observe them in a detached manner.

2    If you do not like the idea of sitting at the bottom of a lake (even an imaginary one), you might prefer to imagine that you are sitting on the bank of a slow-moving river and putting your thoughts on logs floating by. Again, you allow each one 5–7 seconds to pass out of sight, then wait for the next thought.

3    If you are not comfortable with either of the water images, imagine that you are on a clear, open prairie watching puffs of smoke rising from a signal fire. Put your thoughts on to the puffs of smoke, observing them until it is time for the next one.

This kind of meditation should be practised for ten minutes daily for a couple of weeks before you decide if it is right for you. How you decide is simple! After giving it a fair trial, do you feel better *after* doing it than you did before? Do you feel calmer, more centred and in control? If 'yes', continue; if 'no', then maybe you need to try a different meditation.

There are many more benefits to be gained from meditation, and I have been privileged to watch patients blossom as they discover some of their potential. As I mentioned earlier, a person does not necessarily live longer by learning self-help techniques (although sometimes they may do!), but they live better.

I once had a patient, Ben, who had undergone extensive surgery for stomach cancer which had failed to remove all the diseased tissue. When I first met him he was very weak, able to eat only very small amounts, and in despair. Ben was an engineer, used to dealing with facts and figures, and a husband and father. He was also very much used to being in control of things, and had built up a thriving company. When he was referred to me by his GP (very often I appear to be the last resort when a doctor does not want to tell his patient that there is nothing else that can be done) he was very anxious, and desperate to stop the downward spiral in his physical and emotional health.

Because of his practical engineering background, I 'sold' the benefits of meditation to him in terms of blood lactate levels and oxygen consumption facts and figures. Because he was desperate, he agreed to try meditation; normally he would never have entertained anything so 'mystical'. I also supplied him with a relaxation tape and arranged to see him a week later. By the next appointment his colour and posture had improved, and he was clearly beginning to regain his self-control.

After a few weeks of steady progress, he wanted to know what else he could do to improve his lot, and we discussed Lawrence Le Shan's concept of 'finding your own song and singing it'. This meant discovering his creative side and expressing it: 'I've always thought that I would like to paint—I was good at art when I was at school. Maybe I'll buy some paints,' he remarked.

Within weeks he was producing impressive and expressive pictures; he returned to work part-time, and gained weight as his appetite increased. On one visit he asked if he could bring his wife to see me, which I was pleased to agree to, since cancer affects the entire family and not just the patient. I always like to work with the carers as well, and before long I also met his sister. When I asked him if his wife was experiencing any specific problems he said, 'Not problems, exactly. In fact, she's very happy at how well I'm doing because she was told that I would need a lot of care and not to expect much improvement. She just wants to meet you because she says that whenever I go home after

I've been here I'm exhilarated, and she wants to know what's going on!'

When he brought his wife along I explained my approach to her: how I always work towards helping my patients regain some control over their lives, and to live more fully; and about the role of meditation in all this. She admitted that she would never have expected her husband to 'get into anything like this'. He agreed that it was not what he expected when he was referred to me! And whatever the outcome was, he said, he was so pleased to have discovered facets of himself that he had not known existed. Whatever happened, he could accept it.

He had been given a prognosis of steady decline, calling for increased nursing input for about a year. He continued to work part-time, to paint, to put his affairs in order; he regained almost all his weight, enjoyed his food and had very little pain. One Sunday evening I received a phone call from his wife: 'I'm sorry Clare, we have just lost Ben.' His condition had suddenly begun to deteriorate that morning, and he had died peacefully at home after saying his goodbyes; he had had fifteen months of *life* after his surgery.

Before moving on to the more tangible subject of phobias, I would like to share some more of my thoughts on the use of self-help techniques by people with cancer. You have probably frequently been asked by patients, 'Is there anything I can do to help myself?' I have already made my viewpoint clear on the benefits to patients of regaining control with self-help techniques, and improving quality of life, but sometimes these can conflict.

Obviously, a diagnosis of cancer is frequently terrifying, so it is often the case that patients, in their eagerness to 'do something', will take on board all manner of self-help and complementary therapies. It seems to me that often the main reason they do this is that they do not want to die, and will try anything that offers any possibility of avoiding death. This is where the conflict comes in. Presumably the reason for wanting to stay alive is to *live* to enjoy your pursuits, your work, your family and your home, to achieve goals and ambitions and all the things that go to make up life. But if most of your time is taken up with the search for the next sack of organic carrots or a better guru, with your meditation, your relaxation and your visualisation, then what happens to *life*!? Patients can become very good at fighting their cancer, but not so good at living.

I think the aim must be to spend a certain amount of quality time on tackling the illness, but this must be balanced with getting on with living. Patients can forget why they are trying so hard to stay alive, so I always try to restrain the over-eager ones. I was not joking in my Introduction when I said that I recommend my patients to read Terry Pratchett! I believe that 'finding your song and singing it' is also a way of fighting cancer indirectly, and I try to encourage patients to spend less time concentrating on 'the cancer' and more on living more fully.

# 4 Tapping into Their Own Resources

Have you ever heard a song that instantly took you back to a significant time in your life, with all its emotions? Or smelled a scent—someone's aftershave or perfume, new-mown grass, fresh-baked bread—that transported you back to another time and place? Or, perhaps, you were once made ill by something you ate or drank, then could never see, smell or taste it again without feeling ill? Maybe you have a phobia and only have to think about what causes it (spider, snake, needle, bird, high place) or see a photograph of it to break out in a sweat and feel your stomach begin to churn or your pulse to race? This is because our brains are designed to make connections; and usually the more traumatic the circumstances, the more rapidly it happens.

This phenomenon has several different names: behavioural psychology calls it 'stimulus-response'; cognitive psychology refers to it as 'operant conditioning'; in neuro-linguistic programming it is known as **anchoring**. Whatever label you choose to give it, it simply means that sometimes experiencing something (seeing, hearing, smelling, feeling or tasting it), in reality or imagination, automatically and instantly triggers off a physical and/or emotional response. This connection is usually learned accidentally and, in traumatic situations, can be created powerfully and permanently in an instant. Basically, it is designed to make sure that we do not have to go on making the same stupid mistakes ad infinitum. Our ancestor, out looking for food, might have happened upon berries that looked really appealing—colourful and really juicy—so he ate his fill. Unfortunately, they made him desperately ill. The next time he went foraging he had no trouble remembering which shrub caused the problem: the moment he saw it he felt sick, and did not repeat his mistake!

## PHOBIAS

Normally this amazing facility for instant learning is used totally at random, as with a phobia or food aversion, but think for a moment about the possibilities. People who have a phobia *never* forget to activate it! They never walk past a spider, or see a hypodermic, and forget to 'do' their phobia. They never have to think, 'Oh damn, I forgot to be scared— I'll have to go back and do it again!' Imagine learning something so thoroughly, so rapidly and so easily that you *never* forget to do it. How would it be if you could install another response to the anchor that operated just as automatically and instantly? Supposing you could have someone previously needle-phobic look at a hypodermic, and instantly react with a shrug of his shoulders and a 'So what?' reaction. He could have his blood tests, chemotherapy or whatever with indifference.

The good news is—*you can*! Once you realise that many phobias are simply stimulus → response, then you can install 'the antidote'. If you ask a person when she got her phobia, and she replies with some version of 'I've had it all my life', follow the phobia-eradication procedure in this chapter. If, however, she can relate it to a particularly traumatic incident in her life, follow the procedure for dealing with traumas (the trauma cure, Chapter 6). It is possible that when you begin dealing with a patient's simple phobia, she may suddenly remember a traumatic event that initiated it. This has never happened to me; but if it happens to you, 'revert to plan B' and use the trauma cure (p. 127).

If you want to know if someone has a true phobia, either

ask him to image what it is he is phobic about, or begin to talk about it yourself. Either way, if he has a true phobia (as opposed to a mild dislike), his non-verbal signals will tell you. His colour may change, or he may respond with an 'Ooh, no!' or his feet may lift off the floor (then what you are dealing with here is probably a mouse, a spider or a snake phobia). As I explained earlier, the body responds to what the brain is 'playing', and will react as if the threat is real. If you 'test for phobia' in this way, you will realise that phobias live in the mind—and that imagination is sufficient to trigger the phobia. And also to cure it.

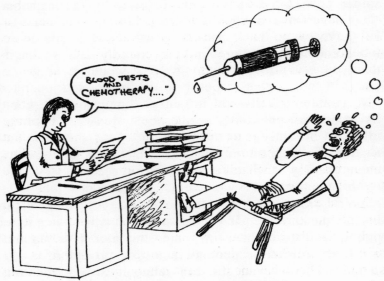

*His imagination never lets him down.*

### The phobia cure

Before launching into the 'instructions', I feel it has to be stressed that you must **act with conviction** throughout the procedure. Until you have succeeded with this routine a few times and gained your confidence, it is natural that you will have doubts—after all, it sounds too simple to be true! But for the sake of your patient, **act as if** it is a commonplace and simple thing to do—do not add to her anxiety by appearing doubtful. This procedure depends on accessing her own positive inner resources, which will be very difficult for her to do if you are ill at ease. Let us take, for example, a patient with a needle-phobia:

1    Ideally, *take your patient out of the problem situation*. You will find it very difficult to get her full attention if, for instance, she is sitting in the chair where she has chemotherapy, surrounded by cannulas and hypodermics. *So take her somewhere neutral and reassure her that you are not going to produce a needle*. You can remind her that she can turn on her phobia without the object of her fear being anywhere around, merely by imagining it, so you do not need to produce the real article to check if the phobia is gone. You will need to be sitting beside or at right angles to her.

2    Ask her what starts the phobic reaction—is it when she sees the needle, feels it touch her skin, or something else? You are trying to discover what the *anchor* is that triggers the response. Typically, the patient will become uncomfortable, displaying some of the symptoms of the fight-or-flight response as she finds the answer.

3    Take careful mental note of her non-verbal signals at this point, so that you can compare them with her non-verbal signals *after* you have fixed the phobia; notice her skin tone, whether her feet are moving, her respiration and so on. Ask her what she is experiencing physically, ensuring that you get 'feel' answers and not 'think' answers. You are looking for responses like, 'My palms are sweaty and my stomach is churning', not 'I am scared.'

If, in reply to your question about what actually initiates the phobic reaction, she says something like, 'It's when I see it coming towards me' or 'It's when it touches my hand,' feed it back to her while gesturing towards the imaginary needle with one hand. It will go something like this: 'So . . . if someone were about to put the needle in your hand', at the same time gesturing towards her hand and looking at it as if you can see the hypodermic (*it helps enormously if you imagine it happening as you are saying it*!). You have just deliberately created an anchor, (I shall refer to this as anchor A) and each time you gesture towards her hand and look at it, it will trigger the phobia. Reassure your patient that 'this is as bad as it gets'.

4   Ask her what she would like to be able to do *when* this is fixed (the presupposition is that the phobia *will* be fixed); feel free to lighten the tension by joking with her about her desired outcome! Usually, with needle-phobia we arrive at a wish to be able to have necessary injections and blood tests with indifference.

5   Ask her if she can imagine doing it now, and watch her reaction again. Point out that she has again turned on her phobia without the needle being present; and that when you have gone through the procedure and she can imagine the needle with complete comfort, presumably she will know that something has changed.

6   The preliminaries completed, you can now start the procedure proper. (This technique is far quicker to actually do than write or read about—my fastest 'cure' was one and a half minutes and the longest thirty-five.) Explain to your patient that you are going to ask her to go through a few memories in her mind's eye—she does not need to tell you what the memories are, so they can be as 'juicy' as she likes. Ask her if it is OK to touch her shoulder briefly while she accesses each memory. (I use the shoulder because it is non-threatening and quite a reassuring gesture.) You can explain that this is simply to establish a 'handle' on the good feelings that go with the memories— deliberately creating another anchor (anchor B), in fact. When someone has a phobia the feelings are usually of loss of control, tension, panic and so on (in claustrophobia there is also often a suffocating sensation), and the memories you are seeking contain the opposite of these

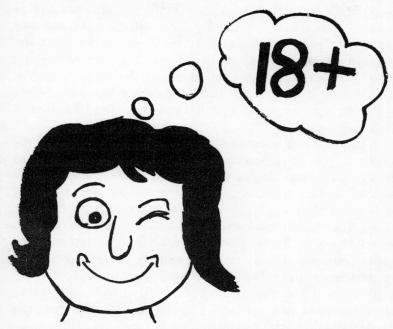

*She is at liberty to keep her thoughts/memories to herself.*

feelings. The routine goes like this . . .

'Remember a time when you felt like 'the bee's knees', a time when you had done something you were *really* pleased with,' you say to her. If necessary you can suggest things like passing her driving test; if you know the patient really well, you may know of some of the more important events in her life. You are looking for a feeling of being in control, of achievement. 'Have you got one? Good! Now, I'd like you to "be there" again. Close your eyes if it is easier, see what you saw, hear what you heard, and above all feel what you felt!'

Use your voice to encourage the feelings, and watch the non-verbal signals on her face to tell you when she has begun to access the good feelings. As soon as you see the change, squeeze her shoulder gently but firmly for around

5–10 seconds to anchor the state. Until you are used to this routine, you may occasionally have difficulty in noticing the subtle non-verbal signals (unless you have done the exercises for sensory acuity in Chapter 2!). If so, just wait a couple of seconds after she has begun the memory before you anchor it! It is much better to anchor too early, when the feeling is coming to a peak, rather than too late when it is fading away.

7   Repeat the procedure exactly, except that this time you ask her to remember a time when she saw or was involved in something so funny that she just 'cracked up' (a relaxed and happy state), and anchor that on the same spot on her shoulder, applying the same pressure.

8   You have now probably done more than enough groundwork to fix the phobia, but I prefer to tap into one more resource before testing. I usually ask my patient to remember a time 'when you had just done something physical and you were feeling pleasantly tired— the sort of tired that you had earned!' This often provokes laughter (especially if I am demonstrating in front of a full class), which just adds to the available resources. Anchor this memory in the same way.

We are approaching the bit that fixes the phobia . . . But first, a recap of how you got to this point:

- You established that the phobia 'lived in her head' by asking your patient to tell you about it, and noticing the non-verbals.
- You discovered the anchor that triggered the phobia (usually something the patient sees), and added your own anchor (A) to it by looking and gesturing at the imaginary needle.
- You decided on the desired outcome—what she would like to be able to do—and established that when she imagined doing it she felt the phobia beginning.
- You decided what the opposite **resource states**—that is, states that brought her feelings of control and relaxation

(point 5)—needed to be and took her through the appropriate memories, anchoring (B) each state. This is a little like having a palette of colours and taking what you need to mix up your chosen shade; or making a stew and adding different seasons until you create the taste you want.

9 *Now*, timing is everything here, and for this to work well it *has* to happen in this order:

*i Say, 'Now', and a split second afterwards—

ii Squeeze her shoulder firmly, on the same spot that you anchored the resource states, and continue to hold it while you gesture and look towards her hand and say, 'Imagine that needle coming towards you.'

Watch your patient's non-verbal signals closely, and you will usually notice a look of puzzlement because she cannot

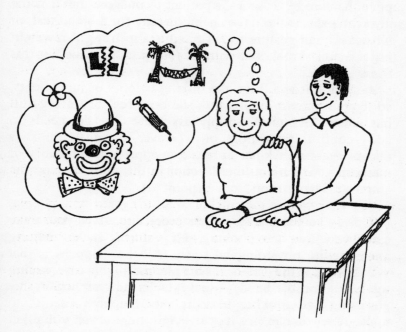

*Imagine that needle coming towards you.*

understand where the phobia has gone. Sometimes she will say something like, 'I can't imagine it,' to which you reply jokingly, 'Oh, go on, I'm sure you can—you could before.' Or she may simply shrug and tell you that she feels nothing; she may think it is weird because it has gone so easily and so painlessly!

10   As soon as you have received confirmation that her reaction is indifference (non-verbal confirmation is really what you are looking for—that is, she remains relaxed and usually fairly still), stop pointing to her hand then let go of her shoulder.

I usually pre-empt the next question, which is often 'It's all very well while I'm sitting here, but what about when it's a real needle?' by reminding her that at the beginning of the exercise she did not need a real needle to turn the phobia on, as the phobia used to live in her mind. I also **future-pace** the cure by asking the patient to imagine that it is the next time she has to have chemotherapy (or a blood test, or whatever) and gesture to her hand again (firing A), watching the non-verbals but without touching the shoulder this time.

As I said, it is a little like mixing colours or ingredients, so if your patient reports that she does feel better but still has some discomfort, simply ask what else she needs to add—control, relaxation, or whatever she may think is necessary—and ask her to recall an appropriate memory or memories, which you then anchor in the same way on the shoulder. Then re-run from * (point 9i).

This is an extremely simple procedure. It works in the same way that the phobia itself worked, by connecting anchors with physiological states. All that happens is that you determine the anchor for the phobia (in this case, seeing the needle on the hand), which you in turn anchor (A) by gesturing and looking towards the imagined needle, to make sure you can **fire** it at the right time. Then you elicit resource states that contain the opposite feelings from those that happen during the phobic reaction, and anchor (B) them so that you can retrieve them at the right time. The final step is to **collapse** these anchors—and it is important to trigger the resource shoulder anchor (B) a split second before you fire the phobia anchor (A), and hold it until you have conformation that there has been a change. In effect you have, at this instant, by firing both anchors together—or 'collapsing' them—fused all these feelings together, and the 'good' ones neutralise the 'bad'. Once done, it does not need to be repeated. And if you wonder how long it will last, think about how long the original anchor (phobia) has lasted.

## Variations on a theme: claustrophobia

For claustrophobia, you can gesture to imaginary lift doors closing, or a radiotherapy shell (more about this in a moment) coming towards your patient's face, or comment on the click as the shell is fastened down to the 'bed' in radiotherapy. Among the resource memories for claustrophobia that I have found useful to ask for is a memory of when the patient was out in the countryside or on the coast on a cool, fresh day, encouraging her to remember how far she could see, the temperature of the air on her face and any scents in the air. These were the sort of resources that I used with one patient in a large hospital with several floors, who needed to be taken in a wheelchair to various departments for tests but, because of her claustrophobia, was unable to travel in the lift.

I have countless case histories that I could quote to illustrate the usefulness of this technique, as there is never a working day that passes when I do not use it, either on its own or in conjunction with the trauma cure (see p. 127). However, I have chosen the following case because I think it might be helpful to illustrate how this technique can also be used very informally.

## *Making use of positive resources: a case history*

A young woman—I will call her Susan—mother of three children, was referred to me by a member of the radiotherapy staff in one of my hospitals. She had a brain tumour and was due to have radiotherapy to her head. For those of you not familiar with this procedure, when a person needs radiotherapy to her head, face, mouth or throat, she has to wear a close-fitting shell encompassing her head during the treatment. This is initially made with plaster of Paris bandages wrapped around the head and face. From this a rigid plastic shell is made, which is placed over the patient's face and head and fastened down to the head-rest on the radiotherapy machine. Sometimes a tongue-depressor has also to be used. The object of this exercise is to mark on the mould the areas to be treated repeatedly, in order to ensure accuracy each time. Obviously, when treating such a delicate area it is important that no more or less than necessary is affected, and that the patient does not move during treatment. Imagine what this must be like if you are already claustrophobic, as was my patient!

Susan had found the plaster of Paris routine very traumatic, so first of all I 'neutralised' that, using the trauma cure (see Chapter 6), and then dealt with problems she was experiencing with her shell. She was due to have her treatment 'planned', which entailed wearing the shell for some considerable time while X-rays were taken and 'targets' marked on the mould. I took her through the collapsing-anchors routine as described earlier (see p. 66) and, though she became tired and bloated from medication, she made it through her planning and treatment with no particular problems with the shell.

She thought that when she had finished this course of treatment it would all be over, but then discovered that she would have to have radiotherapy to the base of the skull. This would mean her having to have another plaster of Paris mould, more treatment-planning and yet another course of treatment—this time while lying face down. Since there were delays with her initial appointment, she had quite a long time to 'stew'; and no one seemed able to tell her when her treatment would begin and end, so she had no idea when she would be able to resume any semblance of normal life. Eventually she was sent an appointment for her mould-making but, on reaching the hospital, she said she had had enough and could not face any more treatment. At this point a staff member contacted me, and Susan and her husband came to my room, where she repeatedly told me that she was not going to have any more treatment, that she could not face it. She was distressed, as was her husband, so I sent them home and arranged to see them that evening at my home (away from any reminder of 'treatment').

When they arrived I initially avoided any mention of her radiotherapy and deliberately manipulated the conversation, seeking the resource states I thought she needed to get her through the treatment. Although a very courageous young woman, she had temporarily lost her 'fight'; she was tired, emotional and tense. Knowing that she was like a lioness about her children, I thought that would be a fruitful line of approach, so I asked her how they were getting on at school, whether they liked all their teachers. They liked most of them, she replied, but one particular teacher had upset her daughter by blaming her unfairly for something. 'So what did you do about it?' I asked—'I bet you didn't let her get away with that!', cranking her up all the time. She went on to tell me how she had gone to the school and confronted the woman. When I saw she was accessing the determination and anger again *I touched her shoulder* and made a comment about the woman sounding a real bitch.

A little later I reminded her that she had promised to let me have the address of the sea-front hotel where they liked to stay out of season. I asked her what the weather was like last time they stayed there, what were the best places to visit and, when she was showing enthusiasm, *I touched her shoulder*, at the same time remarking that it sounded just the place to escape to for a few days.

We talked a little longer; then *I touched her shoulder again* and said, 'We really must talk about your treatment', to which she replied, 'I'll just have to get on with it. After all, I've come this far and I won't let it beat me now!' The object of the exercise had been to give my patient her choices back. She desperately wanted to live, but had become so unresourceful that she was unable to have the treatment. Linking her own inner resources to the treatment enabled her to choose whether she went ahead or not, where previously she had felt that she had no choice at all.

Next day I stayed with her while she had her mould made, and she was fine; and at one point during planning she fell asleep. Several weeks later she and her husband came to visit me, on their way home from an appointment with the consultant, with the news that the scans showed no trace of disease.

The phobia cure I have just described is my accidental adaptation of one of the earliest neuro-linguistic programming techniques, 'collapsing anchors', created by Richard Bandler and John Grinder. We have anchors created and fired in us all the time. They can be visual, auditory, kinesthetic, olfactory (to do with smell) or gustatory (taste)—advertising directors have this off to a fine art—and they cause us to have all manner of feelings, often without our realising why. In addition, once you are aware of the power of anchors and how they work, you can create your own in order to turn on resourceful states in any situation. If you have *ever* felt in control, confident, relaxed, focused and so on in *any* situation, you can link those feelings to any other situation.

In this chapter I have explained only how to use kinesthetic ('feeling') anchors in dealing with phobias but, as I have said, anchors can be created using any or all of our other senses. You could, for instance, tap your pen on the desk at the moment your patient is accessing his resourceful memory, rather than squeezing his shoulder. I have found that using the shoulder to anchor resource states works perfectly for the vast majority of patients, but if this is undesirable for any reason you can anchor using a sound each time, or touch the person's arm or hand.

Recently I was teaching a group of nurses about managing stress in palliative care. When I had finished explaining about kinesthetic anchors and how to use them, I asked for a volunteer with a phobia who would allow me to demonstrate the technique on her. One of the class immediately responded, and joined me at the front of the room. She had a spider-phobia, she said. I asked if it would be OK to touch her shoulder, to which she replied, 'No, I can't bear anyone touching my neck or shoulders!' This was a little frustrating as I had just spent quite a while explaining the routine, and it seemed a little pointless her volunteering to be a guinea-pig if she was unable to let me use it. There is an adage I try to apply in my life—'Do what you can, with what you have, with where you are'—so I asked if I could use her arm. I got the same reply. 'How about your hand, then?' received the same response. Finally, I asked how it would be if I put my hand, palm down, on the chair arm, and if she then put her hand on top of mine. She was happy with that, so we proceeded to fix her phobia with her setting the resource anchors by squeezing my hand when she was experiencing the 'antidote feelings', and collapsing the anchors when I said, 'Now' and pointed to an imaginary spider. She was very happy to be free of the phobia, but I did suggest that she might seek help with her other problem.

Up to now I have been explaining how *you* can use the power of anchors to help your patients in specific situations, such as with phobias. In addition, it is also possible to *install* anchors in patients to be used in a variety of situations, as needed. After taking you through the steps of this technique I will illustrate how *I* use the power of anchors.

As well as having a multitude of uses in helping patients cope with both their illness and their treatment, anchors can also be incredibly effective in helping you, the health care professional, to remain resourceful.

You can take your patient through the following procedure so that he can instantly become more resourceful in difficult situations: for instance, while waiting for treatment, having radiotherapy or seeing the doctor—in short, at any time that he would like to feel more relaxed and in control.

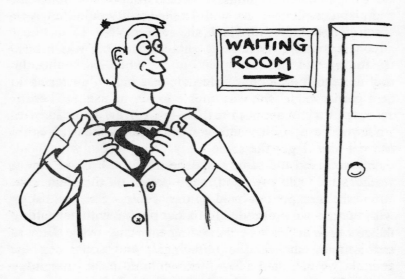

*Hidden resources.*

### Resource anchoring

This technique, like the phobia cure, relies on 'stacking resources'. However, the difference is that the trigger that will bring on the resourceful feelings in this instance is not a specific threat like a needle or a mould; instead, the anchor is in the patient's own control, like a start button, and he or she decides when and where to use it. Another difference is that, unlike the one for the phobia cure, this anchor needs a little reinforcement. As we have seen, in a traumatic situation such as a phobia the mind learns very rapidly; this is why the phobia cure works so quickly. But, because the following technique does not rely on a particular frightening object or event to trigger the resources, a little repetition is needed for it to work really well.

Again, it is a way of transferring *positive resources* from earlier times to whenever they are needed. The patient could do this procedure for himself, but experience has shown me that it is easier to do with someone else guiding him through it, at least initially. Here are the steps:

1 Explain the object of the exercise to your patient: that is, to provide him with a way of immediately becoming more resourceful ('relaxed', 'in control', or however you prefer to describe it). He is going to anchor specific resource states (feelings) in three 'systems' (see p. 38); that is, he will use visual, auditory and kinesthetic 'triggers' to bring on his desired state.

2 He needs, first of all, to decide what feeling or feelings he wishes to use for the purposes of the exercise. This can be either one specific one, such as 'relaxation', or 'confidence' or 'calmness'; or it can be a mixture of states. I often explain this to patients in terms of the palette of colours: you can use straight red paint, or you can add blue to make purple, then add a little white to make yet another shade. Thus, patients can choose 'relaxed and confident', 'relaxed and in control', 'calm and confident', or any permutation of resources.

3 Ask your patient to decide on his anchors for each 'system'. His *visual* one might be an imagined symbol, or something that he could see at a time when he *was* relaxed (or whatever resource, or state, he has chosen). Make sure that he picks something distinctive and memorable. It is not a lot of help if, in times of need, he cannot remember what image he decided upon!

Then, he needs to select an *auditory* anchor. This might be remembering a particular empowering or relaxing tune, or perhaps saying an appropriate word to himself such as 'peace' or 'confidence!' (If he does choose a word to say to himself, it needs to be said in a tone appropriate to that word.)

Finally comes the *kinesthetic* anchor, which needs to be both discreet and discrete. That is, it needs to be something physical or 'feeling', which can be done without drawing

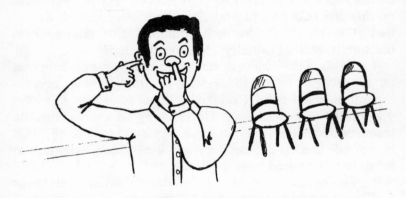

*The kinesthetic anchor **should** be discreet.*

attention to or embarrassing himself; as well as something that is kept solely for the purposes of the anchoring. This could be, for instance, rubbing his thumb and the tip of his little finger together, or, if this is an alien gesture for him, rubbing an earlobe. Having made these preparations, you are ready to take him through the rest of the procedure.

4   For a single resource, such as 'in control', which would be useful during treatment such as radiotherapy, the next step would be to select a memory of a 'bee's knees' or achievement time—just as in the phobia cure. If your patient is mobile, it helps if he can change chairs or take a step forward as he fully associates into the memory—once again remembering as vividly as possible and really

allowing the feeling to develop. It also helps to assume the physical posture appropriate to the feelings—for 'in control' for instance, the head would be up, the shoulders back and the breathing deep and slow. When the feeling begins to diminish, have him return to his original position.

Once your patient is clear about the resource memory to be used, how it feels and how long it takes to fully develop, it is time to begin installing the anchors. This can be done all three at one go, but in practice I find that this is a lot to concentrate on while maintaining the memory vividly; so I will explain how to do it one step at a time.

Decide with your patient which anchor he is going to begin with—visual, auditory or kinesthetic. Then, ask him to relive the resource memory—again, changing position as he begins to do it. This time, *as the resourceful feelings begin to come to a peak*, he installs his selected first anchor. He does this either by saying his word or phrase to himself, or by 'hearing' his tune; or by 'seeing' his symbol or picture; or by making his gesture. As the feelings begin to fade, he ceases firing the anchor and moves back into his first position.

5   He repeats this for the other two anchors, in whatever order he prefers.

6   Now, before testing the anchors, have him change state by asking if he is warm enough, or by commenting on something happening outside the room. Then, ask him to fire each anchor in turn, in the same order in which they were installed, and ask him to notice to what extent the resource state is turned on. Watch his non-verbals carefully, and you should be able to notice changes yourself.

Whether the resulting change in state is judged sufficient or not, it will still strengthen the desired effect if the procedure is repeated. This can be done by using the same memory, other memories with similar attendant feelings or—to return to the palette analogy—by adding a different colour if what is needed is a mixture of resources.

7   It is well worth repeating this procedure several times

to ensure a powerful result and, once your patient has got the idea, he can practise reinforcing it himself if he wishes to. In my experience of this technique, some people respond to one or two of the anchors better than to the others, but initially it is still well worth installing and reinforcing them in all three systems. Eventually it becomes necessary to fire, or think of firing, only one of them for the full effect.

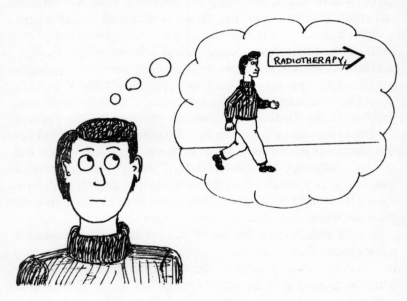

*Think ahead.*

8   It is useful, at this stage, to think of future situations when this resource state would be helpful, and to mentally rehearse them. So, if the targeted situation is having chemotherapy, have your patient decide at what point it would be useful to use his anchors. Will it be when he sits in the chair for his treatment? Or might it be seeing the face of the doctor or nurse who administers the drugs? It might be when he has a feeling—his stomach beginning to churn or his hands becoming clammy. Or it might be something

that he hears, like his name being called or his own internal dialogue saying, 'Oh, no!'

9    Ask your patient to mentally go through this situation. When he gets to the signal that he has chosen as the point at which to bring his resources into play, he must fire all three anchors. If he does this a few times, then this signal will begin to fire his anchors automatically; so, for instance, the sound of his name being called will instantly bring on relaxation (or whatever the chosen resources(s) was (were).

Before I go on to summarise, it may be helpful in understanding what has gone before if I share with you a couple of examples of how *I* use resource anchors. The only difference between my resource anchors and the ones that you will be able to help your patients create is that I very deliberately created mine at the time when the good things were happening, rather than from memories of the events at a later date. This goes back to the 'filters' I discussed in Chapter 1. Because I am well aware of the power of anchors, I have a 'filter' that 'flags up' events, as they are happening, to use as resources later.

If you ever happen to be in one of my classes or at a presentation I give, you may notice that just before I get to my feet I glance at my left knee, and then begin to grin! This is a result of anchors I installed when I had just completed a hugely successful presentation. It was the first time I had spoken in front of such a large audience—around eighty people—and I had been terrified. However, several things got me through. One was a quote from novelist Ian St James: 'If you want to do anything in life, bite off more than you can chew. Then chew like mad!' Another was a cultivated ability to *act as if* I did this sort of thing all the time. Most importantly, I had spent countless hours in planning the content, the visual aids and the pacing of my presentation.

I got rapturous applause and a standing ovation as I sat down. I knew that this was too good an opportunity to miss, so I looked at the notes in my hands, heard the applause and my own internal voice exclaiming 'yes!' (you know the kind of 'yes!', when you punch the air?), and, as I rested my hands on my lap, I pressed my left index finger down on my knee. Later on, I reinforced it by going over the memory again and repeating the anchoring. Now, if ever I am daunted by an audience, or for some reason feel not in my best state to teach, I have only to glance at my left knee to instantly re-create those feelings.

Another set of anchors I use to bring on instant exhilaration; as you can probably imagine, this is useful in all manner of contexts! This one was created as I was driving along a country lane, a short cut to one of my hospitals. I was listening to Neil Diamond doing the music from *Jonathan Livingston Seagull*. This is a wonderful and inspiring book, by Richard Bach, of which a film was made with Richard Harris narrating and Neil Diamond's score. Because I love the story and have only to hear Neil Diamond's voice for my spirits to soar, this album is a powerful combination for me! So here I was, driving along this country lane listening to the tape, on a glorious summer day with a clear blue sky, when, as I came round a bend in the road, suddenly before me was the most amazing field of poppies. It was as if the farmer had sown a poppy crop; Monet was talented, but even he could not have captured this glorious scarlet and green field beneath a cornflower sky.

There is one track on that album called 'Transcend, Purify, Glorious' which is sheer buoyancy to me, and it began playing at that moment. The joy was almost unbearable, so I pulled over, got out of the car and sat at the edge of the poppy field. I listened to the song, absorbed the poppy field and clasped my hands together . . . Now, whenever I need exhilaration I only need to hear the song (real or in my head), see poppies (real, imagined or on the poster on my office wall) or clasp my hands.

SUMMARY OF RESOURCE ANCHORING

1   Explain the object of the exercise.

2   Help your patient to decide on the resource(s) he would like to use.

3   Have him decide on the three anchors—visual, auditory and kinesthetic.

4   Ask him to select an appropriate memory and, when he is beginning to relive it, to change position, returning to his initial position as the feelings pass their peak.

5   Repeat the previous step, installing an anchor each time.

6   Help your patient to change state, then to fire his anchors one at a time, noticing which work best.

7   Repeat the procedure several times, to reinforce, with the same or different memories.

8   Future-pace by asking him to think about a time in the near future when it would be useful to have his resource state 'on tap'; and about what would be a good signal to remind him to fire the anchors.

9   Have him do a mental rehearsal of the situation, firing his anchors at the appropriate time.

POINTS TO REMEMBER ABOUT ANCHORING

- Anchoring is a *very* powerful tool and should be used extremely carefully. Ensure that you are clear about the steps before you proceed, and that you follow them closely.

- Watch your patient's non-verbal signals carefully throughout this routine. You should see indications of state change when he fires the anchors, especially when you get to the point of using the anchors in a difficult situation.

- It may take a little time and practice before you, and your patient, gain confidence in using anchoring—but the results are well worth a little persistence.

Anchoring is a tool that gives emotional choices, and I particularly like it for the way in which it uses patients' own resources. If it smacks of manipulation, then it is because it is precisely that; my dictionary defines 'manipulate' as 'deal with skilfully'. It might also seem in some way 'false' to enable a patient to go into a—what has previously been for her—frightening situation, and then for her 'miraculously' to change her emotional state. You may have noticed that many patients go through radiotherapy and chemotherapy with a smile on their faces, regarding them simply as a necessary nuisance—but would you consider their emotional state to be 'false'? They are merely using their own inner resources automatically; and for those of our patients who are unable to do this it does not seem unreasonable, if we can, to show them how to do it.

# 5 More Relaxation Techniques

Relaxation, when you think about it, is the opposite of the fight-or-flight response. There are endless relaxation techniques, some of them concentrating on physical relaxation and others on using mental imagery. In this chapter you will find a variety of techniques, some of them for you to take patients through and others to teach them to use themselves whenever they wish to. As I said earlier, I would rather teach than 'therap' because then I can give my patients some measure of control over their own well-being.

I often use deep relaxation techniques as a first line of defence with patients. I frequently explain the fight-or-flight response in great detail—very much as I discuss it here in Chapter One—and the patient is immensely relieved when she realises why she is getting some of the symptoms she *is* getting. It often helps carers to listen, too, both to help them cope with their own stress and to understand why their loved ones are becoming selfish and irritable, losing their sense of humour and appearing to be very negative.

I then explain how relaxation is an antidote to the fight-or-flight response and can help improve the subject's well-being in many ways. I say something like, 'If you *could* deal with your current problems like you would a tiger, or a man with a club, then after the fight or escape was over you would heave a huge sigh and relax. All the changes that happened when you were threatened would be reversed until the next tiger, which might be months away. Well, deep relaxation is the equivalent of what would happen at the end of the fight or escape. Relaxing lets your mind and body know that there is no immediate threat, so it can "stand at ease" and behave normally.'

I will probably give my patient a tape of the passive progressive relaxation that follows (p. 97) and ask her to make herself comfortable and listen to it twice a day initially, for the fastest results. My directions are fairly permissive: 'Twice a day if you can, but at least once. It does not have to be at the same time each day. Fit the relaxation into your life—not the other way around—but *NEVER* while driving!' I ask her to use it twice daily for the first three weeks, as experience has shown that patients do get more rapid results that way. After that period they can reduce it to once daily, if they wish to. I point out that the object of the exercise is 'not to wait until you get the screaming hab-dabs and *then* try to relax. It is to not get the screaming hab-dabs at all!'

## WHY PRACTISE DEEP RELAXATION?

The benefits to patients of regularly practising deep relaxation are what you would expect from being able to moderate the problems of the fight-or-flight response. Also, if a patient begins regularly practising deep relaxation before beginning a course of chemotherapy, she is less likely to have problems with 'anticipation nausea' later in her treatment. Insomnia is usually the first problem to respond, and appetite, energy, emotional state and physical comfort can all be expected to improve with two weeks of regular practice (and often much more quickly than that).

Recently I visited one patient who was having severe problems because of oesophageal cancer, necessitating surgery. He had eating problems due to lack of appetite, restricted capacity and vomiting. The plan was to treat him with chemotherapy *if* his weight loss could be reversed and his general condition improved.

He complained of a 'lump' in his stomach and was having severe panic attacks throughout the day and night. Within two weeks of starting to practise deep relaxation his panic attacks had ceased. Although he reported waking a couple of times in the night feeling as if an attack was beginning, he 'just rolled over, and it went off'. The 'lump' disappeared and his appetite increased sufficiently for him to begin gaining weight. Other benefits were that he began regaining confidence to be without his wife, so that she could return to work. In addition, her constant headaches had ceased!

One other thing I was able to do to help the couple was to allow them to 'take my name in vain'. You are probably very familiar with this scenario! The patient had undergone major surgery, had been told he would never work again, had been unable to eat or sleep properly, and faced an uncertain future. Until he became ill, he had worked in an environment where everyone knew everyone else. He was quite popular and had lots of friends and acquaintances, and they were not about to desert him and his wife in their hour of need. Consequently, there was a constant stream of phone calls and visitors to the house. Not everyone is sensitive to the needs of patients like this, and some visitors were staying for up to four hours chatting to him.

When someone is feeling desperately ill, the last thing he needs is some well-meaning individual coming along showing their holiday slides and talking for hours about inconsequential things. This patient's visitors all meant well and were trying to show their support. Often people feel embarrassed just 'popping in' for a short while, and feel that they have to stay for a substantial time. Commonly, they fall into one of two traps: either asking pityingly about the patient's state of health, or avoiding the subject like the plague. Either way, it can be very wearing for a polite patient who, realising that his visitor has the best of intentions, is unwilling to ask her to limit or postpone her visit. In circumstances like this, I suggest, people are a lot like food. Some of them are junk food and you do not want too much of them at one time. Others are nourishing and make you feel better, so you need more of them. So I give the patient permission to say: 'The woman from the hospital [me, of course] has been to see me, and she says it is essential for me to do my relaxation, so I must ask visitors to stay only half an hour [avoid afternoons/ only come on Mondays (or whatever he wants to tell them)]'. He can then choose to tell different things to different people, as he wishes; however, I do tell patients to keep a note of what they have said to whom!

I once had a hospital patient constantly surrounded by kindly, caring visitors who did not seem to notice that her eyes were glazing over and her smile was becoming fixed as she desperately tried to stay awake. Being well brought up and a lovely girl, she too had found herself unable to ask visitors to go. Her health was suffering and she complained to me that she was getting no space to do her meditation and relaxation, and was feeling much worse because of this. By the time all her many visitors had gone she was exhausted and upset—this is one drawback of open visiting hours. It was at this point that I came up with the analogy of junk food and nourishing food, and patients being able to 'blame' me for visitors not being able to stay for a long time. I reinforced it with a note stuck on the TV at the foot of this patient's bed: 'You are not here for *their* benefit!' 'Taking your name in vain' might be a useful service to offer your patients if you feel they are too kind, unselfish or unassertive to put their own well-being before their visitors' feelings.

## Some precautions

The body reacts to what is playing in the head (as we saw in Chapter 1); so if you play relaxing 'movies' in the mind, the body is likely to relax. Many of the commercial relaxation tapes rely on this for their effect. They conjure up images of walks on beaches and the sound of waves breaking on the shore; or scenes of mountain streams complete with sound effects. The more senses you can bring into an imaginary

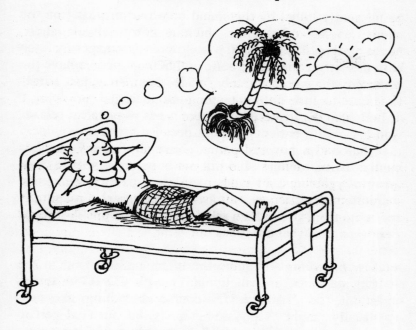

*The body reacts to our own internal movies.*

scene, the more readily the body will be fooled into believing that it is actually happening now.

I have reservations about imposing my idea of heaven on to another person—one man's meat can definitely be another's poison in this area! My own relaxation tape is distributed in hundreds every year, and has been given away in vast quantities to launch a new drug in Europe. I do not get to meet many of the people who use my tape, so I am very careful about the effect I might have on them. I once worked with a person who had been witness to her husband and child drowning in the sea while they were on holiday; amongst other things, she desperately needed her stress levels reduced. Imagine what effect some well-meaning soul could produce by giving her one of the tapes that asks you to imagine that 'you are on a warm sandy beach, being gently lulled by the sound of waves breaking on the shore . . .' My own tape, which is comparatively short, has a progressive relaxation followed by imagery of the patient's own choosing. I believe that most people have the resources they need already inside them; they just sometimes need a little help in tapping into them.

I am also very careful about the types of physical relaxation I use with patients. Again, because my tape is widely distributed I have to make sure, above all, that my methods cannot harm anyone. I work with patients with a vast array of problems, all types of cancer, cardiovascular and respiratory diseases, as well as with people who are simply suffering from stress. So a relaxation method that is safe for *everyone* to use cannot focus on:

- *deep breathing*—imagine the effect on someone in the later stages of mesothelioma, or with COAD or severe asthma, for instance. Of course, breathing exercises (usually taught by physiotherapists) have a vital part to play in the management of these conditions, but not as relaxation exercises. At one of my hospitals I hold relaxation sessions for patients on the respiratory diseases unit, avoiding any mention of deep breathing during the exercise. The ward staff often laugh about how different the patients are after a fifteen-minute session. There is an improvement in breathing, colour and emotional state. Neither can a relaxation method that is safe for everyone focus on:

- *clenching muscles*—for a variety of reasons. I have found that people who come to me for help are usually experts in tensing muscles and do not need to practise! The idea behind this type of exercise is to clench the muscles, then relax and become aware of the difference. But what mostly happens is that people simply revert to the tense state they were in in the first place. The main reasons why I rarely use muscle-clenching exercises, and never on a tape, are that they are likely to increase any pain the

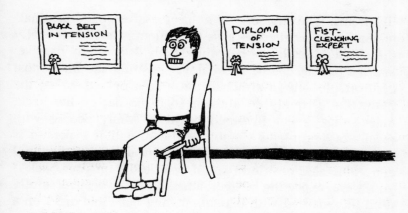

*Will it **really** help, to practise what he's already expert in?*

patient already has, and in patients with cardiovascular problems they can actually cause them harm.

The whole purpose of doing any form of relaxation technique with a patient—or, better still, teaching him how to do it for himself—is (fairly obviously) to help him to be more relaxed; to neutralise the effects of the fight-or-flight response, with all the benefits that will bring to his emotional and physical well-being. So (equally obviously) it seems a good idea to avoid methods that will increase tension, pain, anxiety and breathing problems. The benefits can be enormous—a reversal of many of the problems brought about by stress—if relaxation is practised regularly. I have seen great improvements in the quality of life of people willing to take a little time to master the techniques and use them. I often tell them, 'You didn't get that tense overnight—you must have practised for quite a long time! The good news is that it doesn't take as long to get good at relaxing.' Insomnia is often the first thing to improve; appetite, energy, breathing, confidence and interest in life often follow.

I have used all of the relaxation methods in this chapter on patients with a huge variety of health problems, with no ill effects. The first one is a 'progressive' or 'fractional' relaxation—so called because the patient is talked gradually through a relaxation of her whole body. It is totally passive, and the patient can be in whatever position she finds most comfortable—in an armchair, on a sofa or bed, or on the floor. She certainly does not need to be flat on her back, unless that is her favoured position. Many people with respiratory problems cannot lie down, and if a person is very tense and anxious then flat on her back is an unnatural and vulnerable position (would you lie flat on your back if you were expecting a tiger attack?). I have successfully used this method with patients resting head and arms on a pillow on a table in front of them.

### The progressive relaxation exercise

You are about to talk a patient through a relaxation, so here are a few simple guidelines:

- *For the patient*—make sure she is in a position that will be comfortable for approximately 10–15 minutes; that she is warm; that she has used the toilet first if necessary. Ask her to avoid crossing her legs if she can, or she is likely to end up with numb feet after the exercise. Ask her to close her eyes until you tell her to open them, and explain that all she needs to do is listen to your voice and follow your instructions in her mind's eye. Tell her that you will be playing soft background music to help her relax (if you choose to—I always do).
- *For you*—I find that explaining why you are doing the relaxation helps enormously. Men, particularly, often find admitting to stress difficult (of course, this varies with education and culture), so I find explaining the fight-or-flight response in some detail helpful. Patients are often more willing to try relaxation when it is presented in this context. The problem is no longer their perceived weakness, but the fact that they are having to deal with threats

that they cannot tackle physically. This makes 'society' or 'modern life' the problem. Also, I have often found that when a doctor tells a patient that his problem is stress, the patient can misunderstand this to be the same as 'imaginary', or 'all in the mind'; or even think that it implies he is 'not quite right in the head'!

- Pacing is important as you go through this relaxation: you are aiming to give your patient enough time to carry out each instruction. I find it helps if you mentally carry out your own instructions, allowing yourself enough time, before reading out the next one.

- You are aiming to keep the flow going, so do not leave long gaps between speaking.

- Read the words sl . . . ow . . . ly, stretching them out. I have written the 'script' in this apparently peculiar manner to help you until you get the hang of it.

- Keep your voice low, so that your patient has to pay attention to hear you.

- Forget everything you have ever seen on the movies about hypnotists! You need variety in your voice, not monotony; you are not aiming to bore them to sleep!

- Keep music soft; select pieces without an obvious rhythm (you do not want them tapping their feet); avoid favourite classical pieces—they may turn out to be an 'our tune' of some dear departed. There is plenty of soothing 'New Age music' about. I have been using the same piece, 'Tear of the Moon' by Coyote Oldman, for five years now and the vast majority of patients love it (for the stockist, see p. 157).

- If you are holding a group session—and for some reason a group relaxation is very effective—try to keep an eye on all members of the group. If you get the impression that one person is not beginning to relax, slow down a little and aim your next few instructions in his direction.

- Tell them at the outset not to suppress a cough if it happens—that will only make matters worse. If a patient does begin to cough just carry on with the relaxation, a

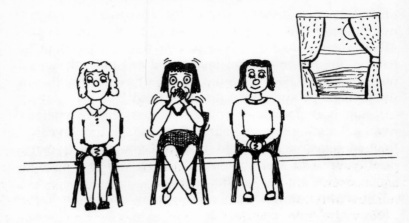

*Suppressing a cough will make matters worse!*

tiny bit more loudly and slowly. If you wait until the patient with the cough has stopped, the rest of the group will lose concentration and the cougher will feel guilty for spoiling the session. So just carry on slowly, and the cougher will catch up.

It is fine to use a script every time, if you want to. In my case it is essential because I am so conditioned to the relaxation that, without the script in my hand, I would be likely to lose my place and grind to a halt (with a silly grin on my face)! Seriously, you might find this hard to imagine at first, but after you have done it with your patients a few times you will find yourself becoming very relaxed while you conduct the session.

At the end of the session, you have several options, depending on circumstances. If patients are in bed you can just leave them to drift off to sleep, should they wish; if they have to do something else after the session, you need to bring them back to an alert state. At the end of your script I have listed some possible endings (p. 99).

I am fully aware that there is a 'prat factor' here; that you will probably feel extremely self-conscious at first. The first time I conducted one of these sessions I just did my best to *act as if* I knew exactly what I was doing, and it worked. I used a script from a book until I decided I could do better myself—now I just do it and enjoy the relaxation (remember 'unconscious competence' from Chapter 2?). If you really are not happy about taking the risk (but I hope you will!), then see p. 158 for details of how you can hear my script on tape. This is it:

Make yourself as comfortable as you can . . . . in whatever position is best for you . . . . and just put everyday thoughts and concerns on one side whilst you enjoy the next few minutes of relaxation. *(long pause)*

Now, I'd like you just to notice how your toes are feeling right now . . . . just notice whether they're tight or re . . . laxed . . . . notice whether they're cool . . . or warm . . . . Just notice how they are feeling . . . . right . . . now . . . .

And in your imagination . . . . however you imagine them is fine . . . I'd like you . . to begin . . to follow those muscles . . . as they go back from your toes . . . . back . . . through the a . . rches . . . and a . . ll the way back . . . . into the hee . . . ls . . . . Now turn a . . ll those muscles loo . . . se; let them grow loo . . se . . . and limp . . . . and la . . . zy . . . . just like a handful of loo . . . se rubber bands.

And a . . s those muscles begin to re . . . lax . . . . let your mind begin to re . . . lax too . . . . Let your mind drift off to pleasant scenes . . . in your imagination . . . .

And now . . . let the re . . . laxation move up into the ankles . . . . and from the ankles . . . . a . . ll the way up to the knees . . . . . The calf muscles begin to grow loo . . se . . . and . . . limp . . . . and la . . zy . . . . . heavy and s . . . o relaxed . . . . All of your tensions are just fa . . . ding away . . . and you're rela . . .xing more with each moment that passes . . . .

Now . . . from the knees . . . . all the way to the hips . . . the long thigh muscles are turning loo . . . se . . . . and limp .... and la .. zy .... ea .. sing off .... and just relaxing now ... And as those muscles re .. lax .... just let go ... a little more ...and gently .... calmly .... easily .... drift into a pleasant state of pea ... ce and relaxation ....

You're relaxing more with each sound that you hear .... Each sou ... nd around you carries you deeper .... and deeper ... and sounder .... into re ... laxation .... And as those muscles relax just dri ... ft all the way ... down dee .. per ... and dee .. per ... into drow .. sy re .. laxation .... Turn all those muscles loo .. se and go dee .. per into re .. lax .. ation.

Now the wave of re .. laxation moves on up ... into the stomach ... and into the solar plexus .... the centre of nervous energy ... Each muscle ... and each nerve ... lets loose its tensions .... relaxing .... and you're drifting down dee .. per ... and dee .. per into re .. laxation ... down dee .. per ...

Up through the ribs .... the muscles re .. lax now ..... Into the broad muscles of the chest .... all the muscles of the chest growing loo .. se ... and limp .... and la .. zy ... and s .. o ... relaxed. All your tensions are fading away ... and you're drifting ... and floating . ; ... drifting ... and floating .... deeper .. and deeper .... into drow .. sy relaxation ..

Into the neck ... the muscles let go now .... All around the neck ... the muscles re .. lax .... just as they re .. lax each night when you're dee .. p in sou .. nd slee .. p .. Turn them a .. ll loo .. se ... and go dee .. per and ... dee .. per into re .. laxation.

Now ... let the re .. lax .. ation start down the back .... from the base of the skull .... to the base of the spine .... Ea .. ch muscle and nerve ... along the spine .... lets loo .. se its tensions .... relaxing .... and you're dri .. fting down dee .. per ..... and dee .. per into drow .. sy ..... com ... fortable relaxtion.

And a wave of re .. laxation spreads out into the broad

muscles of the back . . . . all across the muscles . . . of the back . . . . and a . . ll across the back of the shoulders . . . . Turn loo . . se every muscle . . . . and every nerve . . . of the back . . . . and go dee . . per . . . . a . . nd . . . dee . . per.

Into the shoulders . . . the muscles let go now . . . . . . And from the shoulders . . . . down to the muscles of both arms . . . the upper arm muscles . . . are turning loose . . . . ea . . sing off . . . . . and just relaxing . . . now . . . From the elbows . . . down to the wrists of both arms . . . . the forearm muscles grow limp and la . . zy . . . . . and from the wrists . . . down to the fingertips of both hands . . . . . . each muscle and nerve lets lo . . se its tensions . . . . and you're drifting down dee . . per . . . . . and dee . . per into re . . laxation . . . . .

Into the jaw . . . . the muscles relax . . . . . jaws part-ing slightly . . . . teeth not quite touching . . . . and all around the mouth . . . the muscles re . . lax . . . . and up arou . . nd the nose . . . . each nerve gives way . . . . All around the eyes . . . . the muscles are s . . o heavy . . . . . . and relaxed . . . . even your eyebrows . . . . are relaxing now . . . . .

Across the forehead . . . the muscles smoo . . th out now . . . . . across the top of the head . . . . and down the back of the neck . . . . . Through the temples . . . . and back . . . around the ears . . . All the muscles are loo . . se . . . . . . and limp . . . . and la . . zy . . . . . . just like a handful of loo . .se rubber bands . . . .

You may notice now . . . . . a pleasant sensation . . . . probably in the tips of your toes . . . . . or in your fingers . . . . . a pleasant sensation growing stronger . . . . . and stronger now . . . . as your entire body is being bathed in a pleasant glow of complete . . . . and utter . . . relaxa-tion . . . . Now each muscle . . . and nerve . . . . in your body . . . . is loo . . se . . . limp . . . . . and relaxed . . . . . . .

At this point you can choose whether to say something like, 'And in your own time, you can gradually return to normal, everyday awareness—feeling relaxed, refreshed and alert.' If the situation permits the patient to remain relaxed and drift off to sleep if she wants to, you could end with something like, 'And now, you can remain comfortably drow . . sy and relaxed, drifting into a refreshing sleep if you would like to, until you are ready to awaken.'

If it is necessary to bring the patient to full awareness directly after the session, perhaps for treatment or transport, then the following ending is best:

In a moment I am going to count slowly from 1 to 10, and I would like you to return to normal, everyday awareness by the time I reach 10. You can return to everyday awareness feeling refreshed and relaxed—as if you have had a good long rest; and knowing that you have just done something very positive for your own well-being . . . . One *(starting softly)* . . . two . . . . three . . . . four *(slightly louder and firmer)* . . . . five *(fading out music if you are using it)* . . . . six . . . seven *(louder and firmer as if you mean it!)* . . . . . . eight . . . eyelids beginning to lighten . . . . . . nine . . . eyes opening . . . . . and ten! Back to the here and now . . . have a stretch . . . . .

As I said earlier, I appreciate that initially you may feel very self-conscious talking a patient through this. When, in my classes, I split participants into groups of four to prac- tise this on each other, there is always lively discussion amongst them about who will not go first! However, by the time it gets to the second or third turn the room has become *very* peaceful, and during feedback after the session every- one is pleasantly surprised at how well he or she did. You do not have to do it perfectly for it to work well, and distractions such as outside noise will bother you much more than it will the patients. I once conducted a group relaxation with three male patients who arrived complete with their drips. Half-way through, one of the drips began to bleep because it had been unplugged too long and the battery was getting low. I carried on with the script while reaching around the machine to turn off the bleep. When I had brought them back to normal awareness I asked if the noise had disturbed them; one of them said 'What noise?', and the other two thought it had been an ambulance reversing in the distance. The drip was approximately 18 inches away from two of the men, and three or four feet from the other.

On occasion, someone will fall asleep during the relaxation, but he will nevertheless come back to awareness when you tell him to. If, as sometimes also happens, someone begins to snore, there is no problem as long as the snore

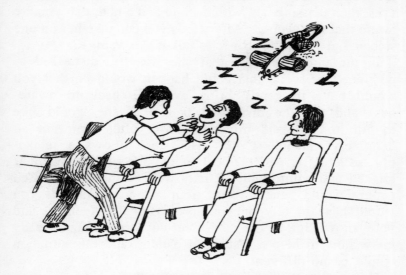

*It may be better all round if you snore quietly.*

remains reasonably soft. But if it begins to sound like a chain-saw, it is a good idea to carry on with the script but gently touch the snorer on the arm to rouse him a little. The worst that will happen is that the rest of the group will collapse into helpless laughter!

Very, very rarely a patient may begin to cry. This is not because you have upset her! It is just that she has been keeping the lid on her emotions and becoming relaxed releases what was there. What you do in these circumstances depends on a number of factors. If you are holding a group relaxation, watch the person who is upset and judge whether she will be OK if you continue. Normally she will; I have never had to halt a group session because of a patient becoming upset, and in total I have probably taken many more than a thousand patients through this relaxation. I have had a patient become upset only perhaps two or three times, and then he or she shed just a tear or two before relaxing again. If your patient opens her eyes, then reassure her, with a smile and a nod, that you are aware that she is upset. Afterwards you can take her on one side and give her the chance to talk if she wants to.

In the unlikely event that she was too distressed to continue, the worst that could happen would be that you would have to gently bring everyone back to awareness and ask the distressed patient if she would like to talk to someone privately. More often than not an extremely valuable group discussion follows a relaxation session, as patients feel more in control as well as relaxed and comfortable. It may well be that a distressed patient would benefit from group support. For this you would have to rely on your professional judgement and your knowledge of the individual concerned. You already know how to help a distressed patient, and this situation would be no different.

If you were taking just one patient through a relaxation when this happened, it would probably be best to take the opportunity to allow him to talk to you about what is on his mind—you could always do the exercise later. Before leaving this subject, though, I must repeat that this is extremely unlikely to occur, so please do not be put off doing something so beneficial for your patients because of the minimal risk that one of them might feel relaxed enough to release some of their pent-up tension.

### *The four-anchor exercise*

As I remarked earlier when discussing relaxation tapes, I am very hesitant to impose *my* idea of relaxing imagery on to my patients. Not only might it be entirely inappropriate, but I believe that the vast majority of people have a storehouse of images already in their memory waiting to be used. The more vivid the image that is used for relaxation, the more effective it will be; and a person is much more likely to be able to conjure up a memory than create something mentally from my description.

The exercise that I am about to describe combines relaxation with *anchoring*, which you became familiar with in Chapter 4. It makes use of a series of the patient's own pleasant memories plus the relaxation these bring (remember: what is playing in our internal cinema *is* 'reality'), and then anchors this resourceful state. After doing the exercise a few times, the brain connects the good feelings with the anchors—which in this case is gently touching the tip of each finger in turn to the tip of the thumb. This is a portable, gentle and very pleasant exercise that takes between 5 and 10 minutes to do. And when the anchors are installed, the exercise can be used as 'first-aid' in times of stress, simply by touching the fingertips in turn. This immediately brings on a calming, 'sigh of relief' feeling.

This immensely effective exercise, taking only minutes, can be used regularly as a stress-reducer, at bedtime as an aid to settling down to sleep, during radiotherapy or chemotherapy, or while waiting for treatment (which can be more stressful than the treatment itself). I also teach it to patients who wish to give up smoking, as it satisfies some of the needs met by smoking such as 'time out', and offers them something to do with their hands as well as being a way of tackling stress. Firing the anchors when the patient is in a particularly difficult situation can often make the difference between coping and not coping.

The exercise can be done one-to-one or in a group; try it

both ways, and see which you prefer. If possible, I like to hold group relaxation sessions, because something very powerful happens when you have a number of people relaxing together. It is a strange phenomenon that even people who have great difficulty relaxing often do better in a group. When running self-hypnosis or relaxation classes I always ask, after the first deep relaxation exercise, who feel that they did not relax deeply enough. Then, for the next exercise I distribute them around the room between people who did relax well. The second time they rarely have a problem! I cannot be sure, but I think that they unconsciously pick up the breathing of the people on either side of them, and as this slows down it leads them into a relaxed state (as discussed in Chapter 2).

This is how you do the four-anchor exercise:

1　Explain to your patient(s) that, just as going over bad memories and worries can create tension in them, so going over pleasant memories can have the opposite effect. You are going to take them through a series of their own pleasant memories and no one else but them needs to know what those memories are, so they can feel free to enjoy themselves! As this is meant to be a *relaxation* exercise, ask that they take responsibility for whichever memories they choose: if they are only able to remember upsetting things, it is better that they do not participate. (I have only ever had one person become upset during this exercise—a nurse who in one of my classes chose, despite the warning, to do the relaxation with the memory of the last time she saw a certain loved one alive.)

2　Before getting into the exercise proper, ask your patients to decide what memories they are going to use, giving them a little time to choose one memory for each of the following four categories. Tell them not to fall into the trap of swapping memories midstream because they cannot decide which is best. If they are lucky enough to have lots of good memories, then they can use different ones each time they do the exercise! The categories are:

i   A time when they had been doing something physical, and they were pleasantly tired afterwards—'that sort of tired that you have earned'.

ii  A time (which might overlap with memory i) when they had a loving, affectionate or warm experience—whatever that may mean to them. This might be a physical experience with a partner, a happy time with a special friend, or with a child or a pet.

iii The nicest compliment they remember receiving. This is very often the most difficult memory to find, or at least to admit to! Many people can immediately remember the last time someone said something hurtful to them, but cannot ever recall receiving a compliment. This is possibly because we are brought up with 'rules' about 'not blowing our own trumpet' and notions such as 'pride comes before a fall.' You may need to give patients *permission* to remember compliments at this point. I often use a little manipulation here, with a remark like, 'When someone pays you a compliment it is usually because they want to make you feel good; it's as if they were giving you a gift to please you. If someone gave you a present would you go, "Oh, I don't think much of that!" and throw it in the bin?' Most patients respond with, 'Of course I wouldn't!' Once they have agreed that a compliment is like a gift, it is fine to accept and enjoy it.

iv  A beautiful place, or somewhere they have felt particularly content and relaxed—it may even be their own sitting-room.

3   When everyone taking part has a memory for each category, explain that you are going to talk them through each memory in turn, helping them to fill in the details to make it more 'real'. Also explain that you are going to ask them to touch the tips of their fingers on one hand gently, in turn, to the tip of their thumb—one for each memory. This is so that, after doing the exercise a few times, they only

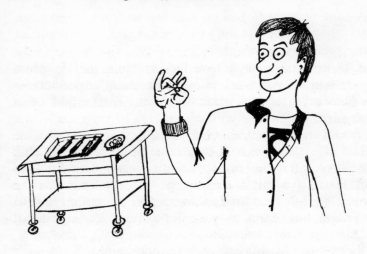

*Your resources at your fingertips.*

have to touch their fingertips to their thumb in order to immediately feel more resourceful.

4    It might help at this point if you explain anchoring as I did at the beginning of Chapter 4, by asking if they have ever found that hearing a particular tune brings on certain feelings immediately. Or smelling something . . . perfume, fresh bread, ground coffee or whatever. You can point out that the brain makes these connections all the time without us deliberately doing it, and that this exercise is using that ability for our benefit.

5    Having done all this, which takes far longer to explain than to actually do, you are ready. So ask your patient(s) to get into a comfortable position (sitting or lying), select which hand they are going to use and close their eyes. Tell them if you are going to be using music in the background. What follows is my way of doing it—feel free to use this 'script' verbatim or adapt it as you will. (The language patterns are deliberate here (as with the 'script for the progressive relaxation exercise), learned from my hypnosis training and designed to increase the effectiveness of the relaxation.)

6   The script:

I'd like you gently to touch the tip of your first finger to the tip of your thumb and, as you hold it there, go back to a time when you had been doing something physical and were pleasantly tired as a result . . . that sort of tired that you've earned . . . .

And once you've chosen your memory, begin to fill in the details . . . . . What was the surface beneath you at that time? *(Give them time to access this memory—how long would it take* you *to remember this?)* . . . . What was the scene to the left . . . . *(Allow them time . . .)* . . . . and in front of you . . . . . and to your right . . . .? Remember all the colours . . . . and the textures . . . . .

What were the sounds at that time when you were pleasantly weary . . . . comfortably tired . . . .? And what were the scents . . . .? . . . . What was the temperature of the air on your skin . . . .? . . . . . And how did it feel to be . . . . pleasantly weary . . . . comfortably tired . . . .? How does that feel . . . . .? *(Note change of tense)* . . . . . . . . . . . . . . . . . . . .

Now . . . let that scene fade and move on to your next fingertip . . . . . And as you do so, go back to a loving, affectionate, warm experience . . . . . whatever that means for you . . . . .

And as you do so . . . . begin to fill in the details of that scene . . . . . the surface beneath you . . . . . the scene to the left of you . . . . . . in front . . . . and to the right . . . . .

Remember all the colours . . . . . and the textures . . . . .

What were the scents . . . . and the sounds . . . . . . that you can remember of this loving experience . . . .? The temperature of the air on your skin . . . . . And how did you feel during this loving, warm, affectionate experience . . . .? How does that feel . . .?

Let that scene fade now . . . . and move on to your next fingertip . . . . and as you do so go back to the nicest compliment you remember receiving . . . . .

And begin to fill in the details of that time . . . . the surfaces . . . . . . . The scene all around . . . . with all its colours . . . . . and textures . . . . . .

Remember the scents . . . . and the background sounds . . . . and the temperature of the air on your skin . . . . . . .

And hear the compliment being said all over again . . . . and allow yourself to really accept it . . . and feel good . . . . . . because you are giving a compliment back to the person who paid you one . . . you're showing that you value their opinion . . . . . how does that feel . . . . ?

Allow that scene to fade now . . . . . move on to your last finger while you go back to a place that is special to you . . . . Remember all the little details . . . . . the surface beneath you . . . . the scene all around with all the colours . . . . and the textures . . . . . . What are the scents associated with this place . . . . and the sounds . . . . . ? What was the temperature of the air on your skin . . . . ? And how does it feel to be in that special place . . . . . how does it feel . . . ?

Allow yourself to relax in that special place for a few moments more . . . . . then in your own time gently bring yourself back to the room and open your eyes . . . . *(Fade out the music slowly (if you are using it) and wait quietly while they open their eyes.)*

There are a few more things necessary for the complete success of this relaxation. You must be sure to allow your patient(s) plenty of time to create a good mental image: perhaps 5–10 seconds for visual and auditory images, and a little longer for scents and air temperature and after asking, 'How does that feel . . . ?' because it takes us longer to remember these details well. I usually spend around 8–10 minutes on the whole exercise, but it can be done in slightly less if time is short. You may have noticed that at the end of each memory I always ask the question about 'how it feels' in the present tense. I have found that this helps patients to associate into the memory more fully—'How *did* that feel?' is more remote from the memory than 'How *does* that feel?'.

These particular types of memory have been selected for their propensity to bring about a generalised beneficial effect—improved self-esteem, tranquillity, vitality and so on. You could tailor-make your own for specific needs, in the way that I mixed resources in the anchoring exercise to fix phobias (see p. 68). I have found the four-anchor exercise to be very popular.

## A gentle muscle-stretching exercise

When patients have muscle tension problems brought about by stress, where appropriate I will teach them gentle physical exercises. Often tension in the muscles creeps up gradually, coming to the individual's attention only when he gets sore shoulders, a tension headache, a painful jaw or all-over aching; then the pain becomes yet another stressor! I suggest to the patient that he stick a little bit of tape on to his watch or clock to use as a prompt—a little like tying a knot in his handkerchief. The idea is that, each time he glances at his watch and notices the tape, he goes through the following exercise to loosen his muscles. This way, muscle tension never gets a chance to build up to the point of pain and, with practice, the patient gets more used to spotting tension before it causes him a problem. The exercise has him, very gently, stretching (*not clenching*) muscles into the opposite position to the one they go into when in the fight-or-flight response. It can be done with the patient in any position, and I encourage mine to use it while waiting to see the doctor, for treatment, for the ambulance (patients get to do a lot of waiting around).

This is how you do it:

1   Ask your patient to close his eyes and, if appropriate to his condition, to take a couple of slow, deep breaths—it helps if he can imagine that he is breathing in through his

navel—then exhale in a long sigh through the mouth. (For the rest of the exercise, also, you can miss out the deep breaths if there are contra-indications.) Again, give him plenty of time to complete each step.

2   The script:

Now, take in another slow breath through your navel whilst pulling your jaws apart inside your barely closed lips; and let the breath out as you let your jaw just relax. Breathe at your own pace as you notice the looseness in your mouth and jaw.

In your own time, take in another breath through your navel whilst you pull your shoulders down, away from your ears; then as you let your shoulders relax just let the breath sigh out . . . . . Breathe at your own comfortable pace as you enjoy the looseness in your shoulders . . . . . and if you wish you can take another deep breath whilst you pull your shoulders down again; then let your breath out and your shoulders relax. Breathe at your own pace and enjoy your loose shoulders . . . . .

Take another long, luxurious breath whilst you stretch your hands, making them as long and as wide as you can . . . . letting them flop down as you allow the breath to sigh out . . . . Then breathe comfortably as you appreciate how good it feels to have loose, floppy hands.

Now this time, as you take in your long breath, push your back against the chairback *(pillows, bed or whatever)* . . . . and as you let the breath sigh out you can stop pushing . . . . and enjoy your loose back as you breathe at your own comfortable pace . . . .

This time, when you take in that long, pleasurable breath, let your knees flop apart . . . . then just relax them when you let the breath out . . . . allowing them to return to their natural position as you breathe at your comfortable pace.

When you take your next deep breath just push your toes gently away from you . . . . and let them flop as you release the breath . . . . Then as you relax and breathe at your normal, comfortable pace you can let your mind spend a little while going over something very pleasing to you . . . perhaps a piece of music . . . . or a favourite flower . . . . or meal . . . . or poem . . . . whatever is most pleasing to you. *(If you know your patient well, you can make suggestions— his favourite fishing/holiday spot, or a celebration meal that he has told you about. People have lots of resources already within them, as you will have discovered if you mentally take notes during your conversations with them. Give your patient a minute or so to fulfil your last request then continue:)* And when you're ready . . . slowly open your eyes . . . . and come back to the room feeling relaxed and refreshed.

I think it is important to have a variety of stress-reducing techniques up your sleeve to offer patients, as different methods suit different people and circumstances. Prevention is always better than cure when dealing with stress, and if your patients have simple techniques like the one I have just described that they can practise regularly, they will begin to regain a measure of control over their own well-being.

## *A calming breathing exercise*

As I said earlier in this chapter, I never use breathing exercises on tape in case the tape is passed on to a patient with respiratory problems. However, there are valuable calming benefits to be gained from this kind of relaxation as, if appropriate to a person's medical condition, such techniques can really 'slow down the system'. This is a very simple one that can be used anywhere, any time that a patient needs to prevent stress rising; again, this is *very* useful while waiting around. The instructions are straightforward:

1   Sit back comfortably, in an upright position in the chair, head up and eyes looking forward; allow your

shoulders to relax naturally. Make sure that you are comfortable in this position.

2   Take 5 slow, deep breaths as you prepare to begin.

3   Begin to breathe in gently for a count of 3, and out easily for another 3. Keep it relaxed and do not try to force the breaths—just gently expand your chest without trying to make the breaths as deep as possible. It may help if you imagine the lungs as being a bucket or a pint glass, filling up from the bottom to one-third, then two-thirds, then to the top, as you count 1, 2 and 3. Imagine emptying the bucket or glass by thirds as you breathe out and count to 3.

Once you have the hang of this exercise, you can go straight into the 3-count wherever you are. It can be done anywhere as it is unobtrusive—after all, most people breathe most of the time!

### *The balloon relaxation exercise*

This exercise is a little more obvious, but it is another mini-relaxation that can be incorporated into a patient's routine. Here are the steps:

1   Relax back into your chair and take a deep breath. Now breathe out fully as if you were a balloon with *all* the

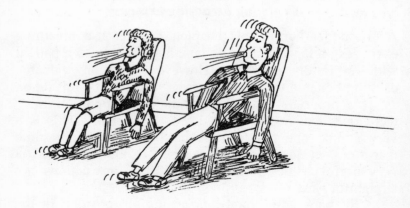

*'Breathe out fully, as if you were a balloon.'*

air escaping. Go down with the deflation . . . then allow your lungs to fill again, without any effort. Concentrate on breathing out all the air, flopping more each time; allow the lungs to refill easily, naturally and effortlessly each time.

2  Continue deflating fully and flopping, then reflating without effort for a couple of minutes—by which time you should feel more physically and mentally relaxed.

Hopefully, in this chapter, you will have found a gentle relaxation to suit any of your patients. The progressive exercise (p. 97) can bring on profound relaxation surprisingly quickly and lends itself well to a tape, so that patients can use it at will (twice daily for two to three weeks can make a major difference to their well-being). Why not consider recording the 'script' so that your patients can reap the benefit even when you are not with them? It is easier than you think, once you get over the initial awkwardness and horror at hearing your own voice!

As I have said, deep relaxation is very powerful in groups, and often the patients you would least expect to are the ones to relax most easily. Often these patients surprise themselves by how readily it happens, and how much better they feel afterwards. In patients with respiratory disease you will usually be able to see their breathing and colour improve during the exercise.

I developed this particular technique initially to use with groups of patients in an out-patients' clinic. They all went through a routine of arriving, having a blood test, seeing the doctor and then waiting for chemotherapy. It is during this waiting time that the tension can mount—and this can lead to increased nausea, higher incidence of anticipation nausea and difficulty in locating veins (which *definitely* cranks up the stress!). Far more preferable is for the patient to begin chemotherapy in a relaxed state. I had to come up with a relaxation that was effective but also fairly quick, so that it would fit in with clinic routine and allow me to accommodate all the patients who wanted to join in.

The progressive relaxation exercise takes less than fifteen minutes which, I think, is about as short as you can make a deep relaxation session. Many of my patients, having gone through the exercise several times with myself or with a tape, are able to relax deeply at will, simply by remembering how it feels when they have been deeply relaxed. You might like to think about ways in which you could use a relatively brief and very powerful relaxation with your patients.

The other relaxation techniques in this chapter are less profound, although the four-anchor exercise (p. 103) gets excellent results and you can expect some grumbles from patients who would prefer to stay in their 'special place' (fourth finger) rather than open their eyes. However, as they are easily learned, the short relaxation methods can play a major role in reducing patients' stress; they can frequently be incorporated into a person's routine to stop tension mounting or used as 'first-aid' in difficult moments, and—above all—they give some control back to the patient, which in itself reduces the stressful feeling of helplessness.

# 6 The Trauma Cure

As you saw with the NLP communication model (diagram 2, p. 16), external events are filtered before we make sense of them. So changing someone's filters will alter his or her internal representation of an event. However, this filtering is not the only thing to happen to our internal 'movies'; as you will learn as you go through the exercises in this chapter, we have many and varied ways of playing them which can also change the ways in which they affect us.

In Chapter 4 I explained how a simple phobia of the 'Oh, I've had it as long as I can remember' variety could be fixed. Now I would like to consider, amongst other things, how conditioned responses that had their origins in traumatic incidents can be dealt with, by changing the way the events were 'filed' in the brain. These too can be many and varied—here are some from my own experiences with patients.

One man could not bring himself to cross the threshold into his consultant's room because, on two previous appointments, the doctor had delivered bad news unexpectedly. An elderly woman was terrified of being discharged home because, just before her admission, she had been attacked in her home by an intruder; she begged me not to make her tell me what he said. Another patient was absolutely terrified to have his second chemotherapy because he had been very ill for several days following his first 'dose'—and this despite assurances that his anti-emetics had now been changed to prevent a recurrence of the problem. I could go on and on, because I deal with a lot of traumatised people, and when people are traumatised their brains make connections very quickly (sometimes called 'one-trial learning'). This is part of our survival instinct—'This hurts, so I won't do it again!'

A classic conditioned response is *anticipation nausea*, which is a notoriously difficult problem to remedy once it has occurred. For those unfamiliar with the term, anticipation nausea can occur when a patient is undergoing chemotherapy which causes nausea and vomiting. The brain makes the connection between the treatment and feeling bad, and this is reinforced with each treatment until—usually around the third session—the response is so strong that the patient will become nauseous *just thinking about* the treatment. It is frustrating for the 'victim', as he is used to the routine and, logically, should not be afraid.

It is far better to try to ensure that this phenomenon does not happen: this can be facilitated by the judicious use of anti-emetics to prevent the patient ever having to experience severe nausea, or by having the patient practise deep relaxation techniques before embarking on his course of chemotherapy. Happily, anticipation nausea is on the decline. Prevention is the ideal, because this reaction to the mere thought of chemotherapy can become so distressing that a patient is driven to refusing potentially life-saving treatment.

This conditioned nausea can become linked in the mind to anything associated with treatment. I dealt with one woman who felt ill when she walked into her own home, because she linked it with returning from hospital still feeling nauseous; she had to throw away her favourite cup and saucer—her husband used to serve her a cup of tea in it on her return home. She could not bear the smell of salad cream—it had been used in the hospital sandwiches; her aged aunt lived on the route to the hospital, and my patient could no longer stand seeing the area. The problem generalised on to so many things that this person was almost permanently nauseous. Another patient suffered severe problems of a similar type. 'It's the trolley that does it!' he started to tell me. I thought he meant the trolley where the syringes for the chemotherapy were laid out, but no. It turned out that he meant the tea-trolley on the ward. When it was wheeled over the carpet strip in the ward doorway all the cups and saucers rattled, and this sound became linked in his mind with feeling sick; so he became ill before he had his treatment—just because the morning coffee came round.

## THE TRAUMA CURE

The trauma cure is another neuro-linguistic programming technique: it can be used to deal with conditioned responses and phobias that began with a specific unpleasant event— such as the problem of anticipation nausea just described. As I said in the last chapter, sometimes I use this technique in conjunction with 'collapsing anchors'. For instance, I was asked to help a female patient who had lost control when her shell and tongue-depressor were put in place ready for radiotherapy. As soon as the mouthpiece was inserted she began to panic and vomit, and the treatment had to be aborted. There was little point in simply attempting to anchor some 'resource states' as described earlier (see p. 78), since the traumatic attempt at treatment the previous day was so fresh in her mind. Each time she thought about having treatment all of the unpleasant memories flooded back and she became panicky and nauseous, so before I anchored resources to her treatment I had to 'neutralise' the memory of what had already happened. This I did, using the method described below, and followed it up with 'collapsing anchors', using the remembered sensation of the tongue-depressor as the first anchor. For resource anchors (again, stacked on a shoulder), I used some of her memories of achievements, of laughing and of wide-open spaces. This took a total of ten minutes, and she was taken for her treatment immediately after. She had no problems whatsoever, and was extremely pleased at being able to put in the tongue-depressor herself. She completed her course of twenty treatments with no further problems.

The trauma cure can be used to make all manner of traumatic memories neutral, freeing the sufferer to move forwards. It changes the way the brain files the unpleasant memories and detaches the event from the feelings associated with it. I recognise that some of life's traumas need to be dealt with over time, to be talked out and come to terms with. However, I also believe that many traumas (the 'one-trial learnings'), such as the disturbing experience with radiotherapy recounted above, that of the elderly woman terrified to return to her previously happy home, the anticipation nausea and so on, need simply to 'unhappen'. By this I do not mean that the patient will experience amnesia of the event; he or she will remember the facts, but almost as if it were a long time ago or as if it happened to someone else.

This procedure is very respectful of the patient's integrity: I have, on occasion, taken someone successfully through the routine without ever having known what exactly had happened to traumatise him or her. The elderly woman afraid to go home was an example of this: she had been simply too embarrassed and distressed to go over the event in detail. After it was 'fixed' she told me what had happened with no difficulty—and then went off to get a cup of tea while she waited for the ambulance to take her home.

The trauma cure is one of the countless techniques to be generated by NLP, and the results are almost magical. In fact, it seems almost too simple and too good to be true, so a little exploration of our thought processes—of how we think—might prove helpful before going through the actual technique.

## Exercises in re-filing memories

*Neuro-linguistic programming is concerned largely with how we think, rather than what we think,* because how we structure our internal representation of events (real or imagined) dictates what physiological and emotional impact those events have. We do not file away 'events'; what we store is a *version* of what happened, after it has been edited (remember the NLP model of communication, p. 16) through the filters of our beliefs and experiences, as well as our emotional state at the time of the event and countless other things.

After our versions of reality have been edited, they are played on our internal cinema; then they are stored away in, if you like, our projection room—ready to play again at a later date (as memories). These 'movies' can be in bright colour, black and white, a mixture of both, sepia, pastels or any variation that the eye can see. They can have a soundtrack, be silent, or be somewhere in between, and the sounds can have all the variations known to the human ear. You may 'hear' the sounds from different directions—the middle of your head, your right ear, your left ear or even your big toe! You may replay your movies as if you were part of the action, seeing what you saw and hearing what you heard; or you may imagine them as a film. You may even remember them as a series of still pictures with a border, or with edges that fade away. Sometimes you may 'project' them outside of your head into different locations. All these distinctions are known in NLP terms as **sub-modalities**. The way we replay these movies (memories) changes the feelings that accompany them.

We have Bandler and Grinder to thank for exploring how we communicate with ourselves (think), and how we can change the way we are doing it if it does not work well for us; or how we can make it even better if it does work. thanks to NLP, we can even find out how someone else who functions in a successful way in a particular field—in teaching, therapy, selling, living happily—does it; how he or she runs his or her programme; then we can use the same programme.

How we replay our memories (and our imaginings) can make a profound difference to the effect they have on us. To help you understand this, try, with a partner, the following exercises in changing auditory and visual sub-modalities.

### Playing with sub-modalities

One of you is designated A, and the other B.

1    A selects *a very pleasant memory*, without letting B know what it is, so it can be as 'juicy' as he likes.

2    As A runs the memory, B asks him to change the sub-modalities of that memory (following the lists on pp. 121–2), one at a time, reminding A to return each sub-modality change back the way it was before doing the next change.

3    A changes the sub-modality of the memory slowly each time, and notices which changes make the most difference to the feelings that come from the memory: which make the memory more or less pleasant, stronger or milder. A tells B of any changes that he is aware of. He notices particularly if a change in one specific sub-modality brings about spontaneous changes in other sub-modalities, either auditory or visual. These are referred to as **critical sub-modalities** or **drivers** and they will have maximum effect on a memory. B keeps a note of the changes for A.

4    Swap around and start again with B as the subject, and go through the above routine again.

5    Change back again. A picks *a mildly unpleasant or annoying memory*—but nothing too traumatic! Now repeat the above procedure with B keeping careful notes of what A notices as you go through the exercise. Notice whether the same sub-modality changes affect both memories—the pleasant and the unpleasant—or do they differ?

6    Swap around again and continue the exercise with B as the subject. Again notice the similarities and differences.

7    Compare notes.

VISUAL SUB-MODALITIES

*associated/disassociated*—ask your partner:
Are you seeing what you saw through your eyes, or are you watching yourself? If you are associated, are you seeing things from a normal angle, or not? If disassociated, what angle are you seeing yourself from?

*number of images*—ask:
Is there one image or more? If more than one, how are you seeing them?

*movement*—ask:
Is it a movie or a still picture? If it is a movie, is it moving at a normal speed, or faster, or slower?

*border*—ask:
Is there a border around the image, or does it fade away at the edges? If it has a border, is this coloured, and how thick is it?

*dimensions*—ask:
Is the image flat or in 3-D?

*shape*—ask:
What shape is the image?

*size*—ask:
How big is the image? Is it panoramic—filling your field of vision? If not, what size is it?

*location*—ask:
How far away is it, and where is it located in space? Show me with your hands.

*colour*—ask:
Is it in colour or black and white?
If it is in colour, are the colours normal—that is, as if you were there? Are they vivid or watercolourish? Or sepia?

*contrast*—ask:
Is the image in sharp contrast, or 'wishy-washy'?

*focus*—ask:
Is it a clear image, or hazy?

*brightness*—ask:
Is the brightness as normal, or darker or lighter?

*proportions*—ask:
  Is everything in the image of normal proportions in relation to everything else? Or is anything bigger or smaller than normal?

Now, go through exactly the same procedure, but asking questions about the auditory sub-modalities, and again taking careful notes for each other. Remember to return each changed sub-modality back to its original state before changing to another.

AUDITORY SUB-MODALITIES
*sound*—ask your partner:
  Is there any sound, or is it completely silent?
*location*—ask:
  Where does the sound come from—inside or outside your head? If it is inside, is it in the middle of your head, in one or both ears, or somewhere else? If it comes from outside, whereabouts does it come from?
*duration*—ask:
  Is it continuous or intermittent?
*volume*—ask:
  How loud is it?
*pitch*—ask:
  Is the sound of normal pitch, or higher or lower?
*inflection*—ask:
  Are any parts louder than you would expect, compared with other parts?
*tempo*—ask:
  Is the soundtrack running at a normal speed, or faster or slower? Does it have any rhythm?

To give you an idea of what use this is, here is an example of how these changes can make a difference very simply. A patient of mine was recently attending for his annual check-up. This young man calls in to see me when he is at the hospital, just for a chat. This time I could tell he had something on his mind, so I asked him if everything was all right. He told me that everything was going really well; he was getting engaged and was working for a company that could offer him a good future. The fly in the ointment was that taking promotion would mean that he would have to give presentations to personnel from other departments in the same company, and also to prospective clients. This filled him with fear, and his non-verbal signals confirmed this. On the occasions when he had tried to address a group of people he had begun to sweat and shake, and had been unable to continue. He felt that everyone was staring at him and judging, he told me.

He was embarrassed at asking me for help, because his problem was not directly related to cancer. But, as I said earlier, I believe in helping people 'find their song and sing it' as an aid to their staying well; and the whole purpose of his going through the surgery and chemotherapy was so that he could *live* fully, so I was happy to help.

So that we could begin with a 'clean slate', I ran through the trauma cure (p. 127) so that his previous distressing experience of public speaking was neutralised. Then, just as in the exercise I have just set out, I asked him questions about his internal images. First, I asked him a bunch of questions about times when he was speaking to a group of friends that he felt comfortable with: were his memories in colour? Were they moving? and so on. I also asked him some of the auditory questions (and in my experience you rarely have to ask all the questions for differences to become apparent). Then I asked him to imagine giving a presentation to his colleagues and his boss. He looked acutely uncomfortable as I took him through the same questions.

It quickly became obvious what the differences were. In the 'friendly' images there was a normal soundtrack, but in the 'threatening' one there was no sound at all. In the first movie all the colours were as real life; but in the second everything was in black and white apart from the heads and faces of the other people, which were in colour, making them stand out. That was why he felt that they were staring and judging—because only the faces, turned towards him, were really obvious.

Once we had gained this information, the next step was easy. I asked him to re-run his threatening movie again, but with all the parts in colour. As he did this his face broke into a broad grin, and he remarked that a soundtrack had suddenly started (so changing colour was *his* 'driver'); it was obvious that he was already feeling much better.

All that remained was to have him, in his imagination, shoot the original 'threatening' image rapidly off into space; then just as rapidly have the new, full-colour version shoot back in to take its place. I had him do that five times—it is like telling the brain, 'Not this . . . *that* instead!' By now he was having a hard time recapturing the old version, which is what I would have expected. I asked him when he would be able to test our work out, and he said, 'Well, I could stand up at the department meeting tomorrow and talk about a project I would like to work on.' I had him mentally run through doing just that, making sure that it was in full colour with soundtrack, and he left in a very optimistic state. Two days later I returned home to find a huge basket of flowers awaiting me, with a card that said, 'I was brilliant! Many thanks.'

I could fill this book demonstrating how you can redirect your internal movies to your advantage. In my stress management classes I spend quite a lot of time teaching participants how to change their emotional state by changing their internal representation of reality—after all, we often have no control over external events and other people's behaviour, but we *can* change how these things affect us. The realisation that we can largely control our emotional state, despite what befalls us, is either one of the most liberating and empowering things that can happen to us, or one of the most threatening! The fact is that once you know how to take responsibility for your own emotional well-being you can no longer blame others for how you feel. (If you would like to know more, see the Bibliography on p. 158).

As a general rule, if we store our memories in colour and are fully associated into them, the feelings from them are strong—and this applies to both good and bad memories. We can re-file them, as you have probably just discovered, and then the feelings change. So it follows that it is not necessarily what happens to us that decides what effect that happening has on us; it is how we 'play' what happens to us. Sometimes people get into the habit of filing their experiences in a way that is disabling for them. This is usually by accident, and they do not realise that they are doing it. Did you know, before you did the exercises in this chapter, how you could affect your feelings simply by 're-directing' your internal movie? We can have much greater control over our emotional state once we get the hang of controlling the way we play reality; and, because the facts of the event are not changed, only the feelings, one reality is just as valid as another.

I once did a home visit to a patient with lung cancer who was experiencing panic attacks. Almost out of the blue she said, 'Does "this stuff" work for depression?' People rarely ask a question like this out of idle curiosity, and with very little prompting she told me that, since the birth of her daughter twenty-five years earlier, she had suffered from depression. Over that time she had consulted several psychiatrists privately and run the gamut of treatments, with no lasting relief.

It is not within my brief (or my expertise!) to take on as a patient someone with such apparent chronic endogenous depression but, when she told me that she got no pleasure from life, curiosity prompted me to ask a few questions. I asked her to remember a happy time. She claimed that she had no happy memories (which is a common claim with the chronically depressed), so I asked her to remember an occasion that should have been happy, had she not been depressed. When she selected the memory of a party when her sister returned from several years abroad, I asked her the same questions about how she remembered it that I have just asked you (see 'Playing with sub-modalities, p. 120).

At first she looked a little perplexed, for which she could be forgiven, as I suppose it does seem a little odd when you have just complained of twenty-five years of depression to be asked if you remember in colour or black and white! She remembered the event in black and white, and as an observer, as if she was watching herself; so her memory of that joyous occasion had absolutely no feelings attached to it. We did this with several similar memories and they were all 'filed' in the same way; so, given that people judge whether memories are good, bad or indifferent by the feelings that are attached to them, her claim to have no happy memories was absolutely true.

Then I asked her to select a mildly sad or depressing memory—and these she remembered in colour and was fully associated into, rather than observing. Imagine what your emotional state would be if you habitually filed your memories—a split second after the event *everything* is just a memory—so that there were no feelings with the good ones and strong feelings from the bad ones. What would your state be, if this went on for years? I then asked her to go back to her 'party' memory and make it colourful, which she did, but with some degree of difficulty. Her posture and skin tone began to change; then, when I told her to associate into the memory, she began to laugh.

I can only hypothesise that she had probably suffered from post-natal depression all those years ago, and during that time of imbalance had slipped into the habit of storing her experiences in that unfortunate manner. The following week I was holding a stress management session for a group of women who had all had breast cancer. Afterwards, I was approached by one of them, who also said she had been depressed for years. I took her through the same routine and discovered that she was doing exactly the same thing with her memories. She was telling me that she could not remember the last time she had enjoyed herself, when her friend interrupted with 'Last Tuesday . . . we laughed until we cried, and you said you couldn't remember when you had last laughed like that!' So, immediately after a happy event, this person was storing it away in her memory with no feelings attached to it. Consequently, when searching for a good memory her inner retrieval system could not find anything filed in the way that good memories are filed.

### The trauma cure step by step

If your patient is still having problems because of something that happened in the past, it is certain that she is remembering it as if she were there again (that is, she is associated into the memory). Ask her to remember the incident briefly again, and you will be able to observe by her non-verbal signals that it still has the power to affect her. In her mind's eye she is seeing what she saw, hearing what she heard and feeling what she felt then. If this were not the case, then the memory would have very little effect (as you have probably discovered). What you are about to do is to have your patient remember the event in a way that will reduce the impact. But you need to build in safeguards to make this a relatively painless procedure, so you utilise the power of anchors again. Your patient is about to recall some potentially traumatic memories, so you need a way of ensuring that she stays in a resourceful state. The procedure goes like this:

1 Establish a **here-and-now anchor** by asking your patient to take careful note of her surroundings: the air temperature, the details of the room, how her back feels against the chair, and so forth. When you can tell that she is really accessing this, squeeze her hand; tell her that if she begins to experience discomfort during the trauma cure, she only has to squeeze your hand and you will squeeze back— and this will trigger the here-and-now feelings. This is sometimes called a **bail-out anchor**.

2   Tell your patient that you are going to ask her to imagine that a fly-on-the-wall camera crew filmed her throughout her 'traumatic incident', and that soon she is going to watch the film on an imaginary cinema screen—that is, she will be watching herself as opposed to 'being there' again. There are two very important points that she must remember: that it was filmed in *black and white*, and that it *starts and ends when she is safe*—that is, it begins before the incident and ends after she is out of the situation and feeling relatively safe (this helps her to set the incident in a larger context by reminding her that she *did* survive). Allow her a little time to decide on the start and finish.

3   Before she begins to 'watch' the traumatic film, ask your patient to imagine that someone has filmed her doing something really mundane or boring—doing the ironing or mowing the lawn are often picked—and ask her to imagine watching a few moments of that on the screen while sitting in the stalls of her imaginary cinema. This serves two purposes, in that it helps her get the hang of the technique while feeling secure and also means that the traumatic event—when 'projected' in the same style—already begins to be re-filed as mundane. It is fine if she wishes to close her eyes throughout this routine.

4   Once she has done this, and established the bail-out anchor, you are ready to go. As I explained in the section on resource anchoring in Chapter 4, it really helps this procedure to go well if you imagine what you are asking your patient to imagine. So tell her that you are both sitting in the stalls watching the screen (gesture with hand to 'screen'), and that you do not need her to tell you what is happening in the film because that will make it harder for her to follow it. Ask her to tell you when she has finished (the presupposition is that *she will finish*), and say that you will tell her what to do next. Remind her that the 'film' is in black and white and that she is seeing herself 'way over there on the screen'. Also remind her about the bail-out anchor—but in my experience patients rarely need it, and only if they

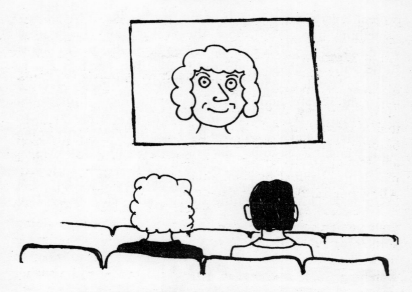

*Both sitting in the stalls, watching the movie . . .*

have associated into the memory again rather than watching it from a distance.

If your patient tells you that she cannot 'see' the film on the screen, ask her to pretend or imagine that she can—it will still have the desired effect. In my experience it is *very* rare for a patient to be unable to do this: when this happens, it is usually caused by the therapist appearing to entertain some doubt, albeit not very much, by saying something like, 'See if you can imagine a film on a screen', or 'Do you think you could imagine that you are going to watch a film?' *I cannot stress too much the importance of acting as if* there is no question that the patient is able to do it. Everyone can imagine pictures at some level; if not, they could not give directions, buy ornaments to match their decor or even recognise their own home. They do not have to be able to do it perfectly for it to work.

5   When she indicates that she has finished, tell her that she is leaving her body in the stalls and going up into the

projectionist's room. Again, help her set the scene; I say something like, 'You know, the projectionist has a little window that he can watch the screen through', and I make a 'little window shape' with my hands. Tell her that she is going to watch exactly the same film—starting and ending when she is safe, and in black and white—but through the projectionist's window. So the screen is 'way down there somewhere', and she will see the back of herself still in the stalls watching the film. This time, ask her to freeze the last frame of the film on the screen when she reaches it, and to tell you when she has done this so that you can tell her what to do next. This is all a little strange, so I reassure her that

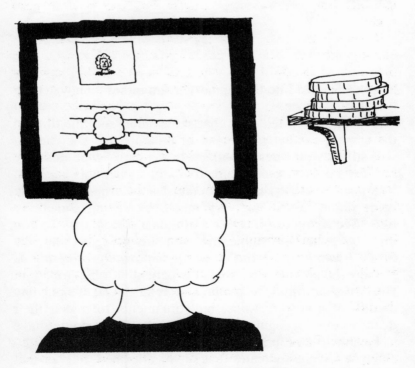

*. . . and now, from the projectionist' room.*

when this bit is over 'we have done most of the work'.

6   When she tells you that she *has* frozen the last frame of the film on the screen, ask her to put herself back into the scene, 'as if you had just finished filming and someone shouted, "Freeze!".'. You are no longer watching, you have just completed filming.' Tell your patient to change it back to colour, although this sometimes happens spontaneously when she imagines actually being there. Now, ask her to imagine that time suddenly goes into reverse and she, and everyone around her, rapidly go through the whole routine *from end to beginning*—everything happens backwards as fast as she can manage it. Ask her to tell you when she reaches the beginning (the presupposition is that *she will reach the beginning*, and to blank the screen. You can reassure her that, although this is tricky at first, it gets easier.

7   Have her run this backwards five times in total, encouraging her to do it as fast as possible. You may notice that, around the third time, she gets slower. If this happens gently tell her, 'Don't stop for the bits you lose, just keep going as fast as you can.' In my experience patients often do lose parts of the film around the third time, and take extra time 'looking for' the bits they lost.

8   When she has finished, 'break state'—that is, bring her back to here and now by making a comment such as, 'Are you warm enough?' or 'The traffic outside is noisy today!', or 'Would you like a drink?' Then ask her to remember the actual traumatic event . . . The usual response is a 'so what?' shrug; or it might simply be that she cannot remember what was so upsetting in the first place. Watch carefully for the non-verbal signals; they always let you know truthfully whether things have changed on the 'inside'.

You will frequently get a behavioural demonstration that changes *have* occurred, although the patient often does not realise that she is supplying it. I was once asked to see a young man who had a terror of needles because of a traumatic incident in his past. It was vital that he have blood tests that day, and he had become almost hysterical at the various attempts to take blood earlier, even though the staff had treated him with kid gloves. When I entered his hospital room he literally bolted up the bed, exclaiming, 'You've not come to take blood have you?'

I calmed him down and told him that I had not come to take blood; and what was more, no one else would, until he felt OK about it. He was very sheepish as he knew that, logically, it was no big deal, and that the tests were important. I said it was OK, and that people in 'not normal' situations often do not act as they normally would; also that, if he followed my instructions, he would be able to have his blood test with no problem. As you can imagine, he was intrigued.

When I asked him to tell me a little about the incident that had caused his phobia he paled and repeatedly swallowed; his breathing became shallow and rapid. I then asked how he felt about his forthcoming blood test, and he told me he could not go through with it. After reassuring him that what he had just done was as bad as this technique gets, I took him through the trauma cure.

When we had finished I asked him to tell me again about 'the incident', which he did in a matter-of-fact way, as if reciting a list of facts. This time there was no change in his non-verbal signals. When I said, 'That's it, you're fixed,' he replied, 'It can't be that easy; I'm off to get the doctor to do my blood test and see if it's worked!' As I said, they often unwittingly give you a behavioural demonstration.

When you have done the trauma cure, there may still be a few things to tidy up. If most of the memory is neutralised, but there is still a part of it which retains some bad feeling, ask your patient to put herself in the memory again, just after the upsetting part, and run that 'clip' rapidly backwards three times—and that usually takes care of it.

SUMMARY OF THE TRAUMA CURE

1 Establish a 'bail out anchor'.

2 Explain to the patient that you are going to ask her to imagine that her traumatic incident was filmed in black and white; beginning and ending when she was safe.

3 Have her rehearse by 'sitting in the stalls' and watching a film of herself doing something mundane.

4 Ask her to run the 'trauma movie' on the screen 'way over there', reminding her about the safe beginning and end, about the film being in black and white, and about the bail-out anchor. Ask her to tell you when she has done it (remember to *act as if*).

5 Now have her float up into the projectionist's room, behind the little window, leaving her body in the stalls; then she watches herself watching exactly the same film—this time freezing it at the last frame and telling you when she has done this.

6 Tell her to put herself, frozen in position, actually in the scene and to change it to colour; then to imagine that time suddenly reverses and everything happens backwards—as rapidly as possible, right to the beginning—then to blank the screen.

7 Have her do this five times in total.

8 Bring her back to 'here and now'.

Needless to say, this requires a certain amount of confidence (or *acting as if*!) on your part. It is well worth your while making an effort to convey, or pretend, total confidence in your patient's ability to carry this technique out. When you have used it successfully once or twice you will no longer have to pretend, as the results can be startling. I derive enormous pleasure in using the trauma cure simply because it enables me to make a huge difference in someone's life, painlessly, respectfully and quickly.

## Anticipation nausea

As I said earlier, this is notoriously difficult to remedy once it has occurred, and can have devasting results. It not only has a severely detrimental effect on a patient's quality of life, but can lead to her refusing treatment. When I came upon my first case of anticipation nausea I did some research and discovered that estimates varied on the extent of the problem—there has been quite a lot of research because the problem is so common and problematical to deal with—but one study showed that up to 61 per cent of patients undergoing chemotherapy suffered from it to some degree. This, happily, has declined, but until nausea as a side-effect of chemotherapy is completely eradicated there will always be sufferers.

Having learned something about neuro-linguistic programming just before I was offered a post in a cancer treatment centre, I knew about the trauma cure, and it seemed to me that anticipation nausea was just another conditioned response. The patient had chemotherapy, which made her ill, and this was reinforced with each treatment. Then she had only to think about coming for treatment, or see/hear/smell something that reminded her of treatment, and the response was triggered. The trauma cure only needed tailoring a little to make it an ideal tool to alleviate anticipating nausea.

All of the instructions already given apply (see p. 127), but the 'movie' is of chemotherapy sessions. Normally, people do not remember all of the details of each of the treatments individually—it's as if they combine into one 'story' particularly if they were all given in the same place by the same staff. Usually you can deal with all the preceding treatments as one event—one trauma. If, however, your patient does for some reason remember every detail of individual treatments, simply deal with them separately, giving them a 'film' each.

As before, the 'film' begins and ends when the patient

feels safe—that is, before she ever came near the hospital, and after her nausea has gone. Have her include as much detail as possible to prevent the problem from generalising on to other aspects of her life (remember the woman who threw away her favourite cup and saucer?).

If you use this technique to deal with all earlier treatments, then as far as the brain is concerned the next treatment is the first. If your patient is undergoing a regime of chemotherapy that has particularly severe side-effects, you could do worse for her than 'wipe out' each treatment before she has to have the next; this way you can prevent cumulative psychological side-effects. Running the trauma cure takes minutes, and gets even quicker as your patient becomes familiar with it. And once she gets the hang of it, and has recovered from the side-effects of her treatment, why not teach her how to do it for herself?

## Using the trauma cure for nausea—a case history

I was approached by the mother of a twenty-eight-year old patient who was undergoing prolonged chemotherapy. He was an only child, still living with his parents, who were very supportive. His mother was extremely concerned as her son was rapidly losing weight because of his inability to eat almost everything she prepared for him. If his weight loss continued, naso-gastric feeding would be the next step. It was becoming an emotive subject because the patient's mother (like many mothers) believed that as long as he was eating he was doing OK, and that she was showing her love for him by preparing his favourite foods and yet he was rejecting them. This will be a familiar scenario to many readers.

It soon became apparent what had happened. He had been given chemotherapy and had gone home feeling nauseous and frail. When his mother, showing her love and knowing how important 'proper meals' were, had presented him with his favourite, his brain connected feeling desperately ill with the meal in front of him, and so it immediately became food to avoid. The next time he came home after treatment, his mother had prepared his second-favourite (he no longer liked his original favourite), and he could not eat this either. And so it carried on, until he had an aversion to *everything* he used to enjoy eating.

I visited him at home and found that, typically, he could not remember each individual treatment or the attempt at a meal that followed it, and so we made the scenario up! Reality is not an essential component of this procedure—I cannot say this too often!—it is how the patient imagines it that is important. We made a list of the meals that he used to enjoy: fish, new potatoes, peas and parsley sauce; steak and kidney pie, carrots, mashed potatoes and gravy; chicken, roast potatoes, cauliflower and gravy, and so on. We included toast, eggs, ice-cream and every other food that he had gone off, in various combinations. As his chemotherapy sessions had all been similar we simply ran through the same 'film' of treatment, but with a different meal waiting for him at home each time. Absolute accuracy was not important— simply, that we included *all* the problem foods.

I received a card the next January from his mum, thanking me for what I had done. She said it 'did her heart good to see him tucking into his Christmas dinner and enjoying every mouthful'.

This technique has a multitude of applications, as I have attempted to illustrate with the examples I gave earlier in this chapter. I have also used the trauma cure successfully with patients who have undergone unpleasant procedures such as a bronchoscopy or surgery, in which the sedation or anaesthesia has been insufficient and they have been left with nightmares and 'flashbacks'.

POINTS TO REMEMBER ABOUT THE TRAUMA CURE

- Before you take your patient through the technique, explain that she will feel differently about the traumatic event when you have finished, and that it may feel a little weird for a while—rather like dropping a brick on your toe and it not hurting! All your previous experience tells you that it should hurt, but now it does not.

- It really helps the procedure along if you imagine the scene as you take your patient through the technique—gesture towards the screen and make a little 'projectionist's window' with your hands.

- Act as if you expect your patient to do what you ask; presuppose by your language that she will go along with you.

- Ensure that she understands that she is watching a film of the traumatic event, but that she is not in it for the first stages. You can help it along by saying something along the lines of 'Watch the film, and you will see someone who looks a lot like you acting your part.'

- Notice her non-verbal signals such as skin tone, breathing and muscle tension while she thinks about the trauma, both before and after you have taken her through the routine. Afterwards, the non-verbal signals will show you that her response to the memory has changed, even before she tells you, and if you do ask her to recount what happened you will find that she tells you in a very matter-of-fact and detached manner.

It must be fairly obvious that I find this technique invaluable and, by now, you are probably already beginning to think of ways in which you could apply it. It must also be clear that I derive a great deal of pleasure from the discovery that I can change my own emotional state by deliberately redirecting my internal movies. I appreciate that this may appear to be a Pollyanna approach to life—almost as if I am refusing to face reality. However, to go back to the women I referred to earlier who were chronically depressed—how 'real' were their memories? They, accidentally, stored their experiences in a way that was detrimental to their emotional and physical well-being. The only difference between my memories and theirs is that I *choose* to store mine in a life-enhancing way, while retaining the facts of my experiences. We all, at times, go through traumas or make mistakes, and we need to learn from them; what we do not need is to be haunted by them.

You may recall the person I referred to in Chapter 1 who became incontinent because of a frightening encounter with doctors in white coats. The trauma cure would have worked in her case but I decided, because her concentration was wavering as a result of her medication, to attempt something simpler first. Before I explain the technique that I used with that patient, try this short experiment.

Are you familiar with the film *Jaws*? Spend a few moments remembering the bit where the shark is stalking the swimmer . . . getting closer and closer. Remember the menacing soundtrack the film-makers use . . . Creepy, isn't it? Now, do that again, but change the backing track to the *Monty Python* or *Muppets* theme, or the 'Birdie song' . . . Ludicrous, isn't it?

The brain registers that silly music is not congruent with threatening images, and re-files them under 'absurd' rather than 'creepy'. Film-makers understand very well how to manipulate our emotions with a judicious mixture of sounds and images. They know that, if they show their advertisements for blue-jeans while playing music that (because of our memories) makes us instantly feel young and vibrant again, we are more likely to buy their product. The next time we go shopping and spot the jeans, we are conditioned to feel good! One of the joys of being aware of how to redirect our inner movies is that we can, if we wish, choose not to be manipulated by ploys such as this. Now that you have experimented a little with re-mixing your internal movies, you will have some idea of what my patient experienced when I helped her deal with her scary memory.

This unfortunate woman, if you remember, had been admitted to hospital for the first time in her life because of breathlessness and haemoptysis. It being a teaching hospital, she had been surrounded by lots of people in white coats, while already in a severely frightened state. In her terror she wet herself, and had subsequently done so again each time she was approached by someone wearing a white coat. Although she had been transferred to another hospital with different (and very kindly) doctors, it continued to be a problem.

When I asked her how the problem had started it was obvious that the memory was still very vivid. I explained that I would like her to remember it again, but in a different way; but before that I would like to know what was the daftest piece of music she could think of. 'The "Birdie Song",' she immediately replied. Then I asked her to run the memory again, but to have that song playing in the background as a soundtrack. She began to grin as I asked her to do it a second time. Then, the third time round, she began to laugh and remarked how stupid it seemed now! Medical staff were a little perplexed afterwards when not only did her incontinence cease, but she grinned at everyone wearing a white coat.

As I said, the trauma cure would also have remedied this problem but, as the actual event had been brief and was traumatic mainly because of her emotional state at that time, it was worth trying something quick and simple. In circumstances such as this, it could also be dealt with as a simple phobia (see Chapter 4), providing the patient is in a fit state to concentrate for the required length of time.

I have attempted in this chapter to give you some tools for dealing with frightening events which, even though they may be from the quite distant past, continue to cause problems in the present and possibly into the future. I would like to reiterate that by the time we have experienced an event it is already a memory: a movie in our heads which has already been unconsciously and unwittingly edited, distorted—even partially deleted—because of our beliefs, earlier experiences, emotional state at the time, and countless other 'filters'. Once you can accept this, you can then help patients to choose how they store *their* memories. As with meditation, gaining control of your own thoughts is probably the best long-term stress-reducer you will ever have.

# 7  Focusing on the Positive

There are several techniques that I use with patients, and teach during my training sessions, that do not fit neatly into the preceding chapters. So here is a mixed bag of things to do with your patients, and things to teach them how to do themselves. The first few are techniques that can help control pain, involving an informal type of self-hypnosis. You need have no worries that, because you are not trained in hypnosis, you can cause any harm with these methods. The very worst that can happen is that *nothing* will happen and you will feel a bit silly!

For these techniques to work you need to be *very* congruent when presenting them to your patients—that is, you have to look, sound and *act as if* you expect them to work. I mentioned this earlier when explaining the trauma cure, and I cannot overstate the importance of 'acting as if'. I appreciate that, at first, it may be difficult to do this, particularly as you are unsure. But, if you can develop the art of appearing confident and relaxed with these techniques, they can be very effective—and almost magical. Often, the more desperate a patient is, the more effective the technique; the brain is looking for an exit from the situation and will accept what appear to be bizarre suggestions, if they are presented with confidence. It helps with congruence if, while you are taking a patient through these routines, you can vividly imagine what you are explaining. This will become clearer as I take you through the methods.

## CHANGE THE PICTURE AND CHANGE THE PAIN

It will probably help you to get the 'flavour' of this method if, before I explain the steps, I describe a brief case history.

The patient was in her late forties and was having severe pain from bony metastases. I was asked to see her almost as a last resort and, as I stood at the nurses' station, I watched her for a little while. She was being put back to bed by two nurses after using a commode, and was obviously in considerable pain although she was receiving diamorphine via a syringe-driver. It also appeared that, quite naturally, she was fearful of any movement. I approached, introduced myself and asked if I could sit down (I always ask permission, as this is the patient's only bit of territory while in hospital, and I am a guest in his or her space).

'I have been asked to come and see you to find a way to make you more comfortable,' I said. (The presupposition is that there *is* a way; this is where the congruence begins, and the brain starts to recognise a possible exit from the situation.) She said that she hoped I could help, as she was at her wits' end and would do anything for some relief. She told me that the pain was most severe in her right hip, describing it as agony. 'Suppose I didn't speak English and you had to draw me a picture to explain your problem—what colour would you make the pain?' I asked. (I am constantly surprised at how amenable patients are to answering my strange questions; I have found that, as long as I am totally congruent, they will play along.) She, looking perplexed, said, 'Red, it's definitely red!'

Then I asked her what size and texture it was; she replied that it was about the size of two hands and was spiky. My next question was 'And what colour will it be when it has gone [spot the presupposition!]? What colour is totally comfortable?' She decided on pale blue; the size and texture was to be of a cotton-wool ball. Then, resting my hand very lightly on her hip to focus her attention on the area, I said, 'OK, now change it from red to pale blue.' She could not manage that, she said, so I replied with, 'Well, begin by changing it to purple, then; that will be half-way. Tell me when you've done it [another presupposition].' After about half a minute had passed she said, 'I've done that.'

'Now you've got the hang of it! Now change it all the way to pale blue and tell me when you've done it.'

About another thirty seconds passed, and then she opened her eyes and exclaimed, 'It's gone!' After telling her I would be back the following day to see her, and reminding her that she now knew what to do, I left. The next day I returned to the ward to find her bed empty, so I went to the nurses' station for an update on her condition. I was told that she had had a good night's sleep and that they had been able to reduce her diamorphine. Then, as I spoke to the nurses, I saw my patient *walk* back into the ward (she had been to the toilet) and climb on to her bed completely unaided. The continuing improvement in her physical and emotional well-being was demonstrated when she returned to the hospital for her next course of chemotherapy—she had had a perm—she walked cheerfully back on to the ward waving and calling out, 'I'm back!'

Yes, this does sound a little like the *Twilight Zone*, but I have used this same technique countless times, and to good effect. I am not totally sure how or why it works, but it could be a combination of things. When a person is suffering severe pain, he or she can become locked in the 'pain cycle' (see p. 9). I think that, by acting with total assurance and confidence that you are going to do something that will help (and not that you are merely going to *try* to) you affect the fear and tension elements of the cycle. Remember, the brain is seeking a way out and will accept almost anything offered with congruence.

This technique has a definite hypnotic element, in that the patient is being asked to enter an altered state of awareness by 'going inside' (hypnotists refer to this light trance state as 'downtime') and making a picture of the pain; as I said in the Introduction, you do not need a swinging watch to induce hypnosis. Once the patient has given you his representation of 'pain' and 'comfort', it follows that if he can change the picture he will be able to change the pain.

I do not think anyone knows for certain how hypnosis can stop pain. Some suggest that in some way it increases endorphins, but Hilgard and Hilgard in *Hypnosis in the Relief of Pain* argue that, if this were the case, naloxone would nullify the effects of the hypnosis; and this does not happen. It is almost as if you have entered an agreement with the unconscious mind; and I have found that, almost invariably, if the patient can come up with pictures of his pain, he can gain some measure of control over it. Although I am not sure how it works, I *am* sure that the key is acting as if it *will* work—getting the patient to enter your version of reality for a little while.

I once watched a TV documentary about a Spanish surgeon, Dr Angelo Escudero, who operates on conscious patients without benefit of analgesia. He had preliminary sessions with the patients he was about to operate on during which he (congruently) told them that, so long as they kept saliva in their mouths, they would be totally pain-free. All other medical staff in the operating theatre were members of his family, all behaving *as if* this was completely logical. Needless to say, the patients made sure their mouths stayed moist (wouldn't you?), and they felt no pain.

### The changing-the-picture exercise

The 'colour, texture and size' method just described can be used to change sensations other than pain. I have had patients with feelings of tightness, tingling or churning stomach, and the same principles apply:

1    First and, very definitely, foremost, *act as if you expect it to work*; eliminate tentative words like 'try', 'hope' or 'might' from your vocabulary while doing this!

2    Ask the patient what colour the area of tingling or tightness (or whatever the discomfort may be) is. It may

help if you explain it, as I did with my patient (p. 142), by asking him to imagine that he is making a picture. Ask him what size, texture and weight (if he has described his discomfort as 'dragging' or 'heavy'). Commonly discomfort is red and spiky, or hard, black and heavy 'like coal'.

3   Ask him to decide what colour the tingling will be when it is comfortable (remember the presupposition); and what size, texture, weight and so forth.

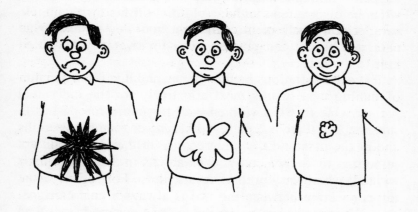

*Tell him to change the picture and change the sensation.*

4   Now tell him to change it from one (uncomfortable) to the other (comfortable). If he cannot manage it in one go, you may have to help him with this. He may have to change it in a couple of steps, like the patient above; or he may have to change the colour first, and then the size. (With patients suffering severe nausea I have often asked them to imagine their stomachs as the surface of a lake during a storm; the desired image is of the storm having passed and the lake's surface becoming calm and smooth like a mill pond.)

Occasionally I have had patients who changed the colour, size and texture of the pain or other sensation, but still had a little discomfort remaining; at that point I tell them: 'Now, shrink it as small as you can . . . then put it outside, on the window-sill.' It helps to have an inventive mind and to be willing to suspend your logic for a while—none of this has *anything* to do with logic! I recently used this technique with a young man who suffered constant chest pain. It had been diagnosed (obviously, it could be dangerous to turn off persistent or severe pain that had not been diagnosed), and would probably resolve itself over the coming months. I took him through the procedure and he burst out laughing when he discovered that he could turn off his own pain. He said, 'I don't believe it—I thought you would have to go and be a hermit and practise yoga for twenty years to be able to do that!'

There are variations on this theme, and it is often a matter of finding what works most effectively for the individual patient. One that has worked well for me in the past is to imagine that there is a path, track, lane or road between the site of the pain and the 'pain centre' in the brain. It is not important to know exactly whereabouts in the brain this is located; wherever you think it is will do. For some reason, my connection between the two is always a dual carriage-way. When you have got an image of your road, you then imagine very deliberately creating a barrier across it: mine is always built of breeze blocks. Build it *very deliberately*, as if you mean it. If the pain returns, either rebuild the barrier even bigger or make your existing barrier more obvious—I whitewash my wall (I did say this has nothing to do with logic!). Another variation is to imagine wires connecting the pain centre and the site of the pain—then to cut the wires.

As I said, these methods make use of 'downtime', the natural light trance state that we all go into many times a day. If it sounds a little far-fetched that hypnosis can have an effect on pain—particularly severe pain, such as that of the woman being given diamorphine—then consider the first fully recorded case of surgery using hypnosis. It took place in France in 1829, and details of it were published in English by Dr John Ellitson in 1843.

A Mme Plantin, aged sixty-four and living in Paris, had a total mastectomy while sitting upright on a chair and chatting to the surgeon, one M. Cloquet. She was prepared for her surgery by her physician, Dr Chapelain, who had hypnotised her on several occasions. While in trance Mme Plantin felt no pain but remained intellectually unimpaired. When in a normal state of awareness, the patient could not bring herself to discuss the surgery and refused to listen to the proposal to operate. However, in trance she was unperturbed. During the entire operation she apparently conversed with the surgeon and his assistant and displayed no sign of pain or movement, no emotion in her voice, and no change in either pulse or respiration. She remained throughout in the same state of 'automatic indifference and passiveness'. Her trance state was maintained over the following two days, during which the wound was cleaned and dressed.

In 1846 James Esdaile, a Scottish surgeon, published his first book *Mesmerism in India, and Its Practical Application in Surgery and Medicine*, in which he reported hundreds of cases of painless operations using hypnosis as anaesthesia. I am not suggesting that the techniques that I have explained above would be adequate for you to begin carrying out surgery (you would need a little more hypnosis training for that), but they can be very effective in appropriate circumstances, and certainly as another way of giving your patients some measure of control over their own well-being.

### Making use of distraction: the 'dead-fish' technique

Sometimes a patient with needle-phobia escapes my attention, and the first I know about her is when she is actually in the chair, about to have the cannula inserted for her chemotherapy. If I am elsewhere in the hospital and have to be 'bleeped', it may be a few minutes before I reach the patient. Contrary to what you might expect, this is often an advantage, because by the time I have arrived the nurses have said, several times, something like 'You'll be OK. Clare's coming!' Contained in this is the presupposition that, when I arrive, I will 'do something' to make things all right. Consequently, when I appear it does not really matter much what I do, as long as I do it with panache and congruence!

One of the things I sometimes do is to take hold of the patient's hand (the one not about to have the cannula in it) and tell her to let it go limp, 'like a dead fish'. This is because it is unlikely that the rest of her muscles will remain rigid if she lets her hand go limp; and this makes it easier for the cannula to go in. I tell her (with complete congruence) that, if she keeps *that* hand floppy, then the other hand will remain perfectly relaxed and comfortable. I keep lifting and dropping her fingers while encouraging and reminding her to let the hand flop and to let me take the

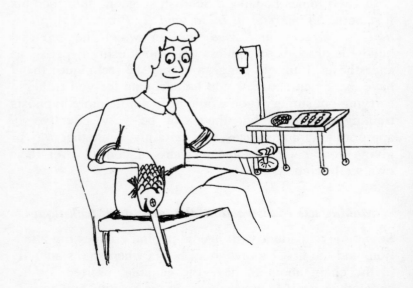

*'Keep the hand floppy, like a dead fish . . .'*

weight. Often the patient does not even realise that the cannula has gone into the other hand.

There is a refinement to this technique, which I use if I have difficulty keeping the patient's attention on her other hand. I go through all of the above, and continue to lift and drop the fingers to encourage floppiness, but I also tell her to start counting backwards from one hundred, in sevens. From time to time I remind her to 'keep the hand floppy like a dead fish'. This is a variation of the 'confusion method' of hypnotic induction. The brain has too much to concentrate on, so the patient goes into 'downtime' (internally focused) and the procedure goes easily.

The first time I ever used this I was asked to sit with a patient who was new to me but not to chemotherapy, while the cannula was inserted, and off the top of my head I went into the dead-fish routine. For the first time ever she experienced no problems having the needle inserted, but afterwards was clearly disgruntled. When I asked her what the trouble was she said, 'That thing with the dead fish!' Perplexed, I responded, 'But your chemotherapy went really well; you never even noticed the needle going in!?' 'Yes, exactly,' she replied, 'but I've had four lots of chemotherapy before this, so why didn't anyone tell me how to do it before now?' I neglected to tell her that I had just made it up, as she might have lost confidence in the technique. Each subsequent time she had chemotherapy she would sit in the chair and make the nurse wait until she had made her other hand into a dead fish; and she had no further difficulties.

## POWER QUESTIONS

The exercise I shall describe next was created by someone who is a most successful motivator and communicator, Anthony Robbins. It is the exercise I mentioned earlier when I referred to techniques to help patients focus on what is good in their life. The **power questions** are not only for people dealing with a life-threatening illness: they are for anyone seeking to change what they focus on. And—I do not apologise for saying this yet again!—what we focus on *is* our reality. Even if an individual has a serious illness, there are probably some things in his life that are still good. I have the 'power questions' stuck on my kitchen wall! To get the best results from this exercise it is important to take a little time over each question, to really consider the answers and allow the feelings to develop.

### *The morning power-questions*

Our life experience is based on what we focus on. The following questions* are designed to cause you to experience more happiness, excitement, pride, gratitude, joy, commitment and love every day of your life. Remember, top-quality questions create a top-quality life. Come up with two or three answers to all of these questions, and feel fully associated. If in any instance you have difficulty discovering an answer, simply change 'am' to 'could be'. Example: 'What could I be happy about in my life now?' So, in the morning, ask yourself:

1  *What am I happy about in my life now?*
   What is it about that that makes me happy? How does it make me feel?
2  *What am I excited about in my life now?*
   What is it about that that makes me excited? How does it make me feel?
3  *What am I proud about in my life now?*
   What is it about that that makes me proud? How does it make me feel?
4  *What am I grateful about in my life now?*
   What is it about that that makes me grateful? How does it make me feel?

*From *Awaken the Giant Within* by Anthony Robbins, Summit Books, 1991.

5  *What am I enjoying most in my life right now?*
   What is it about that that I enjoy. How does it make me feel?
6  *What am I committed to in my life right now?*
   What is it about that that makes me committed? How does it make me feel?
7  *Who do I love? Who loves me?*
   What is it about that that makes me loving? How does it make me feel?

### The evening power questions

1  *What have I given today?*
   In what ways have I been a giver today?
2  *What did I learn today?*
3  *How has today added to the quality of my life?* or *How can I use today as an investment in my future?*

You may decide to tailor this exercise for individual patients, depending on their circumstances. But even a bedridden patient can be a 'giver' by complimenting someone on their hairdo, nightie, smile or whatever. Sometimes a patient may need reminding that *she* can still make a difference . . .

### Have I . . . ?

This exercise is similar to the last one, insofar as it encourages your patient to 'filter' for positive things in his 'reality'. After all, 'reality' is usually a mixture of positive and negative experiences in varying proportions. The intention is not to deny the seriousness of the patient's situation, but to help him focus from time to time on what is positive in his life. This relieves stress and gives him a more balanced view. This is not the same as trying to make him feel better by focusing on the situation of people who are even more seriously ill. 'At least I am not as bad as him' is a very negative way of being positive!

You can either take a patient through this exercise each evening, or copy the questions out for him to use. Once he has used it a few times, he begins to get into the habit of 'filtering' his daily experiences for answers to the questions—and since reality is what you focus on . . .

Ask him, or ask him to ask himself:

*Have I . . .*
>   *. . . seen anything beautiful today?*
>   *. . . tasted anything delicious today?*
>   *. . . smelled anything wonderful today?*
>   *. . . heard anything delightful today?*
>   *. . . touched anything pleasurable today?*

Take a little time to answer these questions, by searching your memory and then reliving as fully as possible each experience. As you go through your days, be alert for experiences you can use as answers to these questions; for instance, if you are near fragrant flowers, take a good long smell and remember it for later. Go out of your way to find things you can use. Listen to music, or for birdsong or for children's laughter. Pay particular attention to the taste of food and drink, to the colours in the sky at sunset, or to the feel of a pet's fur.

As I said, these techniques would not fit neatly into any of the preceding chapters, though they are closely allied to all of the subject-matter. I hope you get the same satisfaction from them as I do, and that they have begun to help you generate your own ideas.

# Conclusion

I have been working with people with cancer for a long time now. When I first came into this field I was fired with an almost missionary zeal to try to gain miraculous remissions for all my patients—and I felt that I had failed if this did not happen. There were times when I wondered why I was putting so much effort in (and over the years I have spent enormous amounts of time and money on training courses and books because of my policy of learning only from the best in their field), if patients died anyway. Of course, I have had many patients who survived and are still surviving; but when one of them died, I felt that I had failed.

Eventually I realised that I was missing the point. And this book has come about from my realisation that it is *making a difference* that is important. What matters is that we help all our patients to live as fully as possible; and there was one patient who was particularly instrumental in my learning this. Since that time I have learned much more, and some of the fruits of that experience are what you have been reading.

At that time I was, for light relief, conducting evening classes in self-hypnosis and, as you would expect, each group included one or two people with cancer. When Barbara and her husband, Barry, enrolled on the first evening, my heart sank. She was obviously very ill, in much discomfort, and with her right arm completely useless and heavy with oedema. I could not imagine how I was going to get her sufficiently comfortable to relax enough to learn the techniques. I think this was the first time that I realised that, the more distressed the patient, the more his or her mind will accept an 'exit'. We supported her with lots of cushions, and she took to self-hypnosis like a duck to water.

Barry was so eager that other people dealing with cancer should enjoy the benefit of his wife's experiences that he wrote a letter to me, expressly to use to 'spread the word'. What follows is taken from that letter:

Dear Clare,

As you know, Barbara was afraid of hypnosis in the early days, through an experience she had many years ago. However, when we started attending your self-hypnosis classes she quickly became reassured about the techniques you were using and realised that she was in charge of what was happening. As a result she very quickly became adept at putting herself into hypnosis. Originally Barbara was using self-hypnosis to help her relax and sleep more easily. In fact she was able to stop taking one to two sleeping pills each night, and just had one occasionally.

But as the cancer and consequent pain progressed she began to use self-hypnosis for pain control. This enabled us to reduce the dosage of morphine to a nominal amount—from 160mg twice daily to 60mg once a day; and diamorphine from 5–10mg every four hours to 5mg occasionally. We found that we sometimes had to use the diamorphine during the night when she would be awakened by severe pain and was unable to turn it off by self-hypnosis.

As Barbara's illness rapidly progressed and the pain increased she found it difficult to turn the pain off. At your suggestion we came over to see you and you taught her the technique of having a 'pain volume control' which she could turn down. This technique she used with great success! It was used successfully in various situations—for example, when out in restaurants, in the car, whilst at the hospital awaiting treatment, and visiting or being visited by friends. [*When she was having to take high dosages of analgesics she was unable to sustain any social life because of drowsiness, lack of concentration and slurred speech.*] Barbara also used the self-hypnosis to make her arm feel lighter; to feel cool when she was very hot; to imagine icicles around the area being treated and re-treated with radiotherapy. We were warned that these areas would probably blister but, I believe as a result of the self-hypnosis, this did not occur!

In the last three weeks of Barbara's life she seemed to be using the self-hypnosis as a life-extending tool; for example, she slowed her breathing down to a remarkable degree. The nurses attending her commented on this! [*This was also reported to me by her nurse who, on several occasions, thought that Barbara had died because of the apparent cessation of her breathing. She used to unnerve the nurses by opening her eyes, taking a breath and smiling at them.*] During this period Barbara told me that she kept drifting into a beautiful valley filled with flowers and very vivid colours. There were people there, and it was all very peaceful and tranquil. She realised that she was being called away but said she wasn't ready yet to go. She said that I shouldn't be afraid of death as it was a beautiful place and she wasn't afraid of going there.

She said that she would like to talk to a family friend, a church minister, but when I told her that he was away on holiday she said that she'd wait until he came back. On his return he immediately visited us. We had a long talk with him about the good times, and some of the sad ones; and Barbara told us that she was ready to go and said her goodbyes.

She died very peacefully the following day after listening to her relaxation tapes. Barbara had been fighting cancer for three and a half years. In February the doctors said she had a matter of days, and she died seven months later.

Barry goes on to tell how the self-hypnosis helped to keep him calm enough to take care of Barbara's dressings right up to the end, with both of them resourceful enough to discuss funeral arrangements and make plans for the family.

I consider it a privilege to have been allowed into the lives of this very special couple. I have never come across two more open-hearted, honest, devoted and humorous human beings. Barry wrote the letter because he believed he owed *me* a great deal. I will never be able to repay my debt to patients such as these for what I learned from this experience about the importance and rewards of simply making a difference.

# Useful addresses

The Anglo-American Book Company Ltd, Underwood, St Clears, Carmarthen, Dyfed SA33 4NE; phone/fax 0994 230400. Mail order books and audio/videotapes on NLP, psychotherapy and hypnosis; also, a postal NLP video library.

The Proudfoot School of Hypnosis, Blinking Sike, Eastfield Business Park, Scarborough YO11 3YT; phone 0723 585960, fax 0723 585959. Mail order books on NLP, hypnosis and psychotherapy; also, provider of training courses in these disciplines and supplier in UK of music tapes by Coyote Oldman.

Both of the above provide a helpful and speedy service.

The Association of Neuro-Linguistic Programming (ANLP), 27 Maury Road, London N16 7BP, can supply a list of NLP trainers in Britain. They also hold conferences with a wide variety of presenters from the NLP field.

# Further reading

Andreas, Connirae (1989). *Heart of the Mind*, Real People Press.

Bandler, Richard (1985). *Using Your Brain for a Change*, Real People Press.

Bandler, Richard, and MacDonald, Will (1988). *An Insider's Guide to Sub-Modalities*, Meta Publications.

Brooks, Michael (1989). *Instant Rapport*, Warner Books.

Davis, H., Eshelman, E., and McKay, M. (1988). *The Relaxation and Stress Reduction Workbook*, New Harbinger Publications.

Dilts, R., Halbom, T., and Smith, S. (1990). *Beliefs: Pathways to Health and Well-Being*, Metamorphous Press.

Hilgard, E. R., and Hilgard, J. R. (1984). *Hypnosis in the Relief of Pain*, rev. ed., W. Kaufman.

Kostere, Kim, and Malatesta, Linda (1989). *Get the Results You Want*, Metamorphous Press.

Le Shan, Lawrence (1983). *How to Meditate*, Turnstone Press.

Lewis, Byron, and Pucelik, Frank (1990). *The Magic of NLP Demystified*, Metamorphous Press.

O'Connor, Joseph, and Seymour, John (1993). *Introducing Neuro-Linguistic Programming*, Harper Collins.

AUDIO TAPE

Rushworth, Clare. *Progressive Relaxation and Stress Management*, £4 (inc. p. & p., from 85 Storrs Hill Road, Ossett, W. Yorkshire WF5 0DA.

# Index